2008

To my very good Patient
Denise Maurer:

Thank you for the
regard & trust
you've shown in
my care through
the years.

MY
CHILDREN
ARE
NEARSIGHTED
TOO

FIRST EDITION

Designed by Meridith Feldman

Note from authors: Throughout the book we've referred to eye professionals as "eye doctors." There is understandably confusion among patients, since there is more than one type of provider of vision care and not all of them are doctors. Most likely your child's vision care will involve optometrists, opticians and ophthalmologists. Each plays an important and unique role in maintaining a child's clear vision. We recommend working with the eye professional who treats your child (and you) with respect in a professional and comprehensive manner. Let your instinct be your guide, not the vision provider's degree, insurance plan participation or their office location. In our office we are privileged to work with all three types of eye professionals, since each fulfills specific needs for our patients.

Thank you to Asian America TV, Paragon Vision Sciences, Wink Productions, Inc., All Sports Photo, and Shutterstock® Images for their photographs.

www.MyChildrenAreNearsightedToo.com

"A great void in the literature today is a book that is written for parents, and understandable to both children and parents about the management options for nearsightedness (myopia). Such a large – and increasing – segment of the young population are myopic and, as a parent, it is important to understand myopia and what are the best methods of managing this condition with your children. This void has been filled by this text from Dr. Nick Despotidis, along with Drs. Lee and Tannen. They have authored an easy-to-understand guide on the modern methods of managing myopia including an exciting program, entitled corneal reshaping, that allows qualified young people to only wear a vision correction while sleeping at night. A must read for every parent!"

—Edward S. Bennett, OD, MS Ed
Associate Professor - University of Missouri, St. Louis
College of Optometry

"Parents are faced with many dilemmas when raising children, not the least of which is their medical care. Myopia or nearsightedness is one of these medical challenges and Drs. Despotidis, Lee and Tannen have captured many of the parental concerns regarding this condition. I look forward to recommending this educational yet entertaining book to both parents and young people to help them in making informed decisions about the latest in myopia correction options."

—Craig W. Norman, FCLSA
South Bend Clinic
South Bend, IN

"Drs. Despotidis, Lee and Tannen have authored a comprehensive book about nearsightedness and options for its correction, including a technology known as corneal reshaping."

—Jeffrey J. Walline, OD, PhD
Assistant Professor
The Ohio State University, College of Optometry

"Dr. Despotidis has produced a perceptive, interesting and accurate account of the clinical presentation and management of juvenile-onset nearsightedness that will be fully appreciated by parents. I was particularly impressed with Dr. Despotidis' ability to impart clinical wisdom and enthusiasm with reference to a variety of patient case studies including those of his own children."

—Bernard Gilmartin, BSc, PhD, FCOptom, FAAO
  Professor of Optometry - Aston University United Kingdom
  Co-author: Myopia & Nearwork

"For the past 100 years, vision scientists from around the world have struggled with the question on how best to correct nearsightedness. Today, there is a growing body of research indicating that myopia may be controlled in young children through the use of corneal reshaping lenses.

Nearsightedness (myopia) control through corneal reshaping is truly an exciting opportunity for parents and could prove to be one of the most important ocular discoveries in this past century."

—Patrick J. Caroline, FAAO
  Associate Professor - Pacific University, College of Optometry

"Dr. Despotidis has been a leader in the field of corneal reshaping. His latest effort to bring into clear focus the nearsighted (myopic) epidemic which threatens the eyesight of our children is perhaps his greatest contribution to date. In his book *My Children Are Nearsighted Too* he educates and alerts parents to the dangers inherent in lifestyle choices which may be leading to up to half of the current generation of young people becoming nearsighted. To answer this challenge, Dr. Despotidis describes an effective course of action which can lead to a very different clinical outcome - that of healthy eyes and healthy people."

—Cary M. Herzberg, OD, FOAA
  President
  Orthokeratology Academy of America

"This book contains a message of hope. Shortsightedness (myopia) in children can be very frustrating - every eye exam inevitably seems to result in a prescription for stronger glasses. To parents who are desperate to fix this ever increasing problem, there is hope that we are beginning to understand the complex processes involved. Moreover, there is the promise of a relatively new treatment known as corneal reshaping. At a time when experts around the world speak of a "global epidemic of myopia", Dr. Nick Despotidis has produced a very approachable and informative book that will be of great interest to parents and children alike. Put simply, this book offers the hope of a better life for short-sighted kids."

—Dr. Russell Lowe
  Private Practice & Clinical Research, Carlton, Australia

"Written with parental understanding and clinical expertise, Dr. Despotidis and partners Drs. Lee and Tannen, have presented a comprehensive guide to understanding juvenile myopia, ideas for preventing its progression and the cutting-edge treatment options. As a mother of two boys, and a practitioner myself, I agree that corneal reshaping must be considered as a primary treatment modality. I have found that for the proper candidate, this relatively uncomplicated treatment yields remarkable results appreciated by both the young patient and his/her parents."

—Sarah N. Knapp, OD, FAAO
  Private Practice – East Lansing, Michigan

"The unknown is a fear to most, especially parents of children with vision problems. Dr. Despotidis' book provides insight by bringing scientific and clinical knowledge of both vision and vision related problems in a successful way."

—Dr. José M. González-Méijome, OD, PhD
  Auxiliar Professor of Optometry
  University of Minho, Portugal
  Associate Editor-in-Chief, Journal of Optometry

Dedication

To my wife Teresa

If we see the world
through our children's eyes,
we live a blessed life

Acknowledgments

Completing this book has been one of the highlights of my career, due in part to the number of people who graciously gave of themselves.

My wholehearted appreciation to Howard Feldman; you define the word friendship. Without your insight, tenacity and sincere desire to help others this project would not have gotten off the ground. To Barry Tannen, my optometric partner; I'm fortunate to call you a friend and share the "ride" with you. Ivan Lee, your compassion and commitment to excellence inspires me. To their wives, Sandi Tannen and Kim Lee, for their kindness.

To my editors at Wink Productions, Inc., who transformed a manuscript from a bunch of words and facts into a story worth sharing. I'm indebted to you for your sheer inspiration and professionalism.

Brienne Alfano, whose unyielding support and organizational skills make me a better doctor.

Craig Norman, your in-depth review and suggestions were so insightful — you see the forest! PM Hawkins for your never-ending encouragement and assistance; you're the consummate professional. To Professor Bernard Gilmartin for reviewing the manuscript; your brilliance is only overshadowed by your generosity. Dr. Jeffery Walline for your encouragement and expert advice; our profession has evolved due in part by your dedication. To Drs. Michael Lipson, Cary Herzberg, Tara Svatos, Edward Bennett for your support and insight; I'm humbled by your generosity. My sincere appreciation goes to Larry Rosen of LaRocca, Hornik, Rosen, Greenberg & Blaha LLP for their counsel and friendship.

To the parents and patients who lent their reviews; Christine Feldman, Danielle Ring, Dr. Debra Dagavarian-Bonar, Dr. Young-mee Yu Cho, Jennifer Mullen, Jennifer Persichetti, Jesse and Rebecca Wu, Kim Lee, Lisa Jones, Nina Hawkins, Sandy Kossack, Sharanne Papigiotis, Shu Shu Costa, and Sonia Hou--I'm ever grateful. To Amy Zelley for scanning all childhood photos, thank you!

To my parents and sister for their unconditional love and support and to my sons, the underlying inspiration for this book.

To the thousands of patients who generously share their stories on a daily basis with friends and family and to my extraordinary staff; you make every day an *amazing* day!

This book made me wonder what I will do if that day comes.

As an optometrist, I have fit countless children with all varieties of contact lenses, so I was honored when I was asked to write the foreword to this book. However while I was reading this book, I began to think about my own son and experienced it from a mother's perspective. Although he is only a toddler now and has not been diagnosed with myopia, he is at risk. My husband and I both wear glasses, which increase his chances of needing them at some point, too. This book made me wonder what I will do if that day comes? Will I fit him with contact lenses? Will I prescribe bifocal spectacles? How will he feel about wearing glasses or contact lenses? In the end, I realized that I will not know until the time comes. Each child is different and decisions need to be based on interactions with each individual child.

Dr. Despotidis has the same philosophy. I know firsthand how much Dr. D's patients trust and respect him because I have had the pleasure of co-managing his patients when they relocate to Boston. Not surprisingly, they speak very highly of him. I, too, trust and respect Dr. D. As the nearsighted father of two nearsighted children, Dr. D has a personal connection to the condition and his compassion and empathy are conveyed throughout the book.

If you are the parent of a nearsighted child, I invite you to take the time to read this book. The knowledge you gain will help you, together with your eye doctor, to make an educated decision for your own child.

Marjorie J. Rah, O.D., Ph.D., F.A.A.O.
Massachusetts Eye and Ear Infirmary Contact Lens Service
Boston, Massachusetts

Contents

Author Biographies

Appendixes

I'm a Parent Just Like You!

Nicholas Despotidis, OD

Introduction

For over two decades it's been my privilege to be an eye doctor. And in that same time frame it's been my *joy* to be a father. Both roles have moments filled with emotion—some pleasant, some not so pleasant. As an optometrist, one of my most uncomfortable feelings is when I have to tell a mom or dad that their young child needs to wear eyeglasses to see the board in school or watch television at home.

What's even harder is when I have to tell parents that their child's eyesight is getting worse. The look of hurt, guilt and even despair on those parents' faces tells me how concerned they are about the situation.

Parents have many questions; some are asked at the first appointment and others may be formulated in the middle of a sleepless night.

"But he's so young! How can he need eyeglasses?"
"Is it hereditary? Did she get this from me?! "
"What happens as he gets older? Will it get better
  or will it get worse?"
"Will kids make fun of her at school?"
"Is it a disease?"

This book is designed to guide parents through an often confusing, always emotional experience in the life of their child. This book will help you understand how your child's eyesight works, how they use their vision to play and learn, what happens when things go wrong, and most importantly, what the best options are for *your* child. I'm here to help you better understand why your child may need eyeglasses and what can be done now that you know.

I'm here to help because I'm not only an eye doctor,
I'm a parent just like you!

Until recently, many eye doctors thought poor eyesight was genetic and it was blamed on mom or dad. Yet many parents are quick to tell me they have never worn eyeglasses or didn't need them until much later in life. After seeing thousands of patients I sincerely feel that there is more to poor eyesight than simply genetics. Could it be the ever-increasing near work that contributes to the rising number of nearsighted children showing up in my office chair?

And there was another trend; I was prescribing eyeglasses for children at a younger and younger age. With every exam I'd wonder, "Why?!" What was contributing to this phenomenon? Did computer and video games have anything to do with it? What about added hours in front of the television? Could the shift from kids playing outdoors to sitting in front of a digital screen have anything to do with it? Does nutrition play a role? There had to be an explanation!

My questions were still unanswered when something very interesting happened a few years later. This event would also forever change my perspective as an eye doctor. It was the day my son came home with a note from the school nurse:

Mr. and Mrs. Despotidis,

Nicholas is having trouble seeing the board in class. I think he might need glasses. Please have his eyes checked by an eye doctor.

Sincerely,
Mrs. xxxxxxxx
School Nurse

I was stunned! Nicholas was only 7 years old.

Suddenly I was feeling all of the same emotions I witnessed in the parents of my young patients.

"How can my son need eyeglasses? He's only 7 years old!"
"Did he get this from me even though I didn't need
  glasses until I was an adult?"
"It must be my fault."
"How will the other kids treat him at school?"

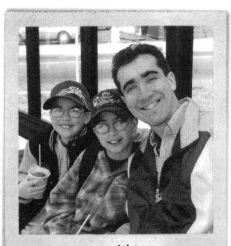

Dr. D. and his sons,
Nicholas and Gregory

A few years later when my second son, Gregory, came home with a similar note it came as less of a surprise. He was also 7 years old.

Watching my own children's eyesight get worse year after year turned my curiosity into action! I changed from being an eye doctor interested in understanding why this was happening to a father dedicated to keeping my sons' eyesight from getting worse and determining what I could do to stop it.

I sincerely hope you will use this book as a resource when questions arise about your child's eyesight. By having answers to those questions, you'll be better prepared to make an educated decision regarding the best care for your child. I've recruited the help of two of the best eye doctors I know, my optometric partners, Barry Tannen and Ivan Lee, to help me simplify the complex topic of eyesight, myopia and options for their improvement.

This book comes from the heart because I'm not only an eye doctor; I'm a parent just like you!

Sincerely,
Nicholas Despotidis, OD, FAAO, FCOVD

My Child Needs Eyeglasses!

Nicholas Despotidis, OD

———————— Part I ————————

Even though I'm an eye doctor,
I'm a father and I was troubled.

When our oldest son Nicholas was 7 years old, I had suspected he was having problems with his vision (I am an eye doctor after all…). I examined him in my office and discovered that he had mild myopia, also called nearsightedness. I prescribed eyeglasses and, in my most sincere doctor voice, told him to wear them only when he had trouble seeing the board in the classroom. He nodded, told me he understood…and promptly lost them. This scenario repeated itself over and over again much to my frustration (I am a father after all…).

After Nicholas lost his first pair of eyeglasses, I simply kept a new pair at home ready to be called into action whenever needed. He only wore them when he wanted to see clearly at a distance. But why did I ask him to limit his use of eyeglasses? Simple, because I believed that wearing eyeglasses all the time would make his eyesight worse (I was wrong about that, but more on that later).

When Nicholas was in the second grade I received the dreaded note from the school nurse. "Nicholas needs to have his eyes examined."

How embarrassing! An eye doctor has to be told his own son needs his eyes checked.

I examined Nicholas again and prescribed stronger eyeglasses, this time as bifocals. No, that was not a typo. Bifocals are the kind of lenses that people over forty wear because their reading vision becomes blurred. But bifocals are often used differently for children than for adults. Children who are nearsighted only need to wear their eyeglasses when they look at things far away because they can see very well up close (hence the term nearsighted). Wearing bifocals allows the child to see through the distance prescription in the top portion when looking at objects far away, but the bottom portion is essentially a clear lens to be used when the child reads or looks at near objects. Just like an adult wearing bifocals, it allows for two different areas of correction without having to remove or change the eyeglasses.

The bifocals didn't work for Nicholas. Not because they weren't made well or weren't the right prescription, but because he had trouble getting used to the different powers within the eyeglasses. No matter how good they are, they can't work when they are left in the case. (Stay tuned for an explanation of the research behind bifocals in Part Three!)

By the fourth grade, Nicholas' nearsightedness had progressed so far he couldn't see the larger letters on the eye chart. Even though I'm an eye doctor and examine children similar to Nicholas every day, I am Nicholas' father and I was troubled because his eyesight was deteriorating rapidly.

The Role of Heredity and Genetics
Did My Child Inherit My Poor Vision?

We all know families (you may even be in one yourself) in which everyone wears eyeglasses, even the children. Nearsightedness or myopia runs in families and it often makes its first appearance in childhood. It's not your imagination; the facts are confirmed by research. If one parent wears eyeglasses for nearsightedness, then the children are more likely to wear eyeglasses than if neither parent wears eyeglasses. And if *both* parents wear eyeglasses, the odds are very likely that the children will wear eyeglasses.[1, 2]

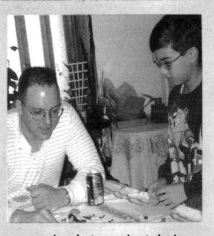

Uncle Chris and Nicholas both wearing glasses

However, just because both parents *don't* wear eyeglasses doesn't mean their children will avoid eyeglasses, too. Unfortunately, more and more children are becoming the first in their family to be diagnosed with myopia even though their parents have never worn eyeglasses. And, the trend in our office is that children need eyeglasses at a younger and younger age.

Why?!

Genetics is definitely a factor in the development of nearsightedness, but by no means is it the only factor and it may not even be the most significant factor. So, what else contributes to the development of myopia?

Environmental Influences

I Don't Wear Eyeglasses. Why Does My Child Need Them?

In addition to heredity, the development of myopia may be influenced by environmental factors such as near work activity. Studies have shown that the more near work children perform, the more likely they will become nearsighted.[3, 4] So, one reason a child's eyesight may start to decline earlier and earlier is the increased amount of near work they perform at younger and younger ages. But as we'll see,

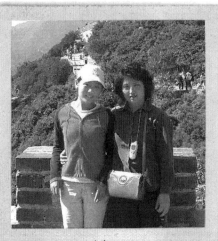

Jessie and her mom, Jie

> **When the school nurse told me that my daughter Jessie was nearsighted, not only was my heart broken, I was also shocked! Both my husband and I have 20/20 vision. I never expected this could happen to my daughter.**
>
> **—Jie**

there are many factors to consider: genetics, environment, family values, even our children's diet!

I've observed that children who start to wear eyeglasses during childhood rapidly become more nearsighted through their school age years. I've found that children who continue their education into college and beyond have stronger prescriptions as they become adults, which has also been noted in scientific articles.[5] Our highly educated students may graduate with the best education, but the poorest eyesight!

As the vision becomes worse, the eyeglasses become thicker. Other than poor appearance, is that really a problem? It is important to realize that higher degrees of myopia mean more than just heavier, thicker eyeglasses. High myopia is also associated with an increased risk of developing eye diseases later in life, like cataracts, glaucoma and retinal diseases.[6-12]

As the degree of myopia increases, so does the effect it has on our children's daily lives. Simple tasks like swimming, bathing, and even walking become an adventure if done without their eyeglasses.

My Child is so Young!
Why Does He Need Eyeglasses?

As our children perform greater amounts of near work, the likelihood they will require eyeglasses increases. When I look back at all the near-vision activities my young children participated in, I cringe! Handheld devices, computer games, video games, and children's books all require near vision. And our children are drawn to these devices at younger and younger ages.

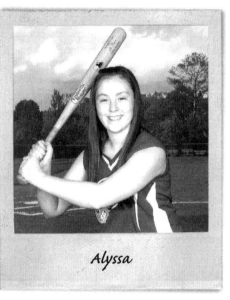

Alyssa

Think back to when you were a child. Without the lure of video and computer games, where did we spend our days? That's right! Outside! Riding bikes, playing ball, climbing trees and skating to a friend's house requires us to use distance vision, not near vision. The activities that occupy our children's time, however require near vision and it could be that they are paying the price with their vision.

Some of us became nearsighted as we entered college. Not only is that the time that our outdoor, distance activities decreased, but our near,

> "Alyssa needed glasses in kindergarten. The following year her prescription got significantly worse. At this time our doctor recommended something called corneal reshaping…I never heard of it, but was interested in any option that would prevent my daughter from having to deal with glasses or contacts during the day.
> —Marykim (mom)

close work increased. We pored over papers, focused on the computer, had our heads in books and many of us started to wear eyeglasses. I am a perfect example; I began to wear eyeglasses in college and my eyesight continued to get worse through optometry school.

In Part Two, Dr. Tannen reminds us that in the earliest stages of human development, it was those with the best distance eyesight, the hunters and gatherers, who lived the longest and were the most prosperous.

Today's society has a different focus. No longer needing to hunt and gather, there are other skills needed for success today. Our children need to have a strong foundation in computers. They need to be well educated. And near work is required for these tasks. The children who perform a greater degree of near work are the ones often praised. The bespectacled Bill Gates is a modern day role model!

Cultural Influences

Does My Heritage Play a Role in My Child's Nearsightedness?

The percentage of people who wear eyeglasses to correct myopia differs greatly among cultures. Take a look at the approximations below for older teenagers. Nepal has a very low prevalence of myopia while in urbanized Eastern Asian cultures, like Taiwan, the incidence of myopia may be over 80%![3, 13]

- 2% Nepal
- 27% United States
- 37% Australia
- 65% Japan
- 73% China
- 83% Taiwan

Why?! Is it simply genetics or is it purely environmental? Looking at the numbers above, it might seem that genetics play the dominant role. That is, until the value different cultures place on academic achievement is also considered.

Some cultures emphasize scholastic achievement and reading more than others. In certain subsets within cultures there is more time spent reading than in others who share the same genetic makeup. For example, one study found that boys in Orthodox Jewish schools are three times more likely to be nearsighted than the boys in general Jewish schools. Now add to the equation that the boys in the Orthodox schools spent as much as 16 hours a day studying![14]

Another report published in the *British Journal of Ophthalmology,* studied 429 people applying to enter the Singapore military. This study found that nearsighted applicants generally had more education than their "clear-seeing" counterparts.[5]

What is important about both of these studies is that the students shared the same genetic makeup, yet the children who did the most near work developed the poorest eyesight.

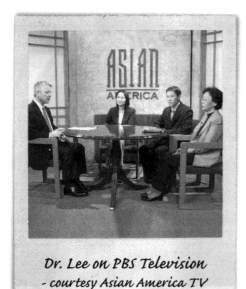

Dr. Lee on PBS Television
- courtesy Asian America TV

In Eastern Asian cultures, academic excellence is highly valued and emphasized. Scholastic excellence is often expected! My partner, Dr. Lee, was interviewed for the PBS television program *Asian America TV* on the topic of "Myopia in Asian Students."[15] When it was asked of the panelists on the program, "Why are children of Asian descent more prone to myopia?" the emphasis placed on academic excellence by Asian parents was the recurring theme.

So, it appears that while genetics has a role, culture and environment play an important role as well.

It Sounds Like an Epidemic!

The prevalence of myopia may be increasing within the United States. But why?

In his book "The World is Flat," author Thomas Friedman describes how events will lead us to compete within a global economy.[16] With improvements in transportation and communication, the world is getting smaller. And the world is already "flat" for our children. The mix of cultural backgrounds that has made our country so strong through the years is evident in classrooms throughout our country.

When I attended college, "perfect" SAT scores were rare. Today, universities have to choose among many applicants with perfect scores![17] In order for our children to compete in this academic "flat world," the pressure is on for them to be computer savvy and test savvy. This requires a great deal of reading and studying!

In countries like China, where the prevalence of myopia is very high, vision scientists are working feverishly to find options that can prevent their most successful students from developing poorer vision. In our increasingly competitive world, our young people's decreasing vision needs our attention.[18]

Helping Our Young People

Are TV, Computer and Video Games Hurting My Child's Eyes?

Parents commonly ask me if too much TV is bad for their children's eyes. If your children sit closer than 8 feet from the television they may be placing unnecessary strain on their eyes. A closer viewing distance requires our children's eyes to actively focus to keep the television clear. A longer viewing distance requires less active focusing. I recommend that children sit at least 8 feet from the television. If your child continues to move closer to the television, despite your instruction to move back, this is often indicative of a vision problem like nearsightedness. If this is the case, a visit to the eye doctor is in order.

The number of hours spent in front of a television or video screen every day is a unique decision that each parent has to make. As with everything else in life, there has to be a balance. Each hour spent in front of a TV or computer screen is one more hour that your child focuses on near objects. Each hour spent playing video games is one less hour playing outside or potentially doing other distance activities.

Nothing seems to absorb my children's attention more than video gaming. I can shout. I can cry. I can jump up and down and flail my arms. They don't move! They don't look up! They don't hear a word! And they can be in this hypnotic state for hours!! What does this have to do with vision? Everything!

Long periods of intense near work have been associated with nearsightedness. Whether the near work causes the nearsightedness has yet to be proven, but there is a connection. It makes sense the demands placed on our children's eyesight may cause their prescription to change.[19] It's not the video game; it's the uninterrupted near viewing for long periods at a time.

The decision to allow your child to play video games is a very personal one. Personally, I recommend no longer than

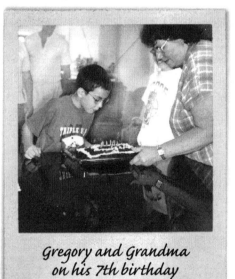

Gregory and Grandma
on his 7th birthday

"My younger son, Gregory, started wearing glasses at seven years old. He often played handheld video games. As his nearsightedness progressed, I limited his video game use."
—Dr. D.

30 minutes of uninterrupted time on any device, followed by a 30 minute break in which they get involved in distance activities, preferably outdoors.

Outdoor activity is very important in helping to keep our children's eyesight from becoming more nearsighted. I recall traveling across the country to hear a noted authority in the field of myopia talk about how to prevent our children's eyesight from getting worse. What do you think he said? "Let your children play outdoors!" I traveled hours and spent days out of the office to hear this message?! As simple (yet out of touch) as that advice seemed at the time, recent research has confirmed his astute recommendation.[20]

My Child Loves to Read in the Car. Is That Bad?

A reading child is a quiet child. I have always loved having my children occupied in the backseat, especially on a long trip. But that was then and this is now.

I ask that my children avoid reading or working up close in the

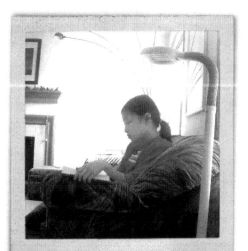

Kelly (G) now reads with better lighting

> In our minds, we blamed ourselves for not taking care of our daughter Kelly; we shouldn't have let her read in the car or play computer games, and provided her with better lighting while reading…After we did all those things her eyesight continued to get worse, she required stronger and thicker eyeglasses each year.
> —Jian (dad)

car. The movement of the car causes the book or object to constantly shift. This requires even greater concentration and this prolonged, often intense focus at near can cause the focusing system to "spasm" or get stuck, a form of sustained adaptation. This is especially true if our children avoid looking up and changing their focus to different distances. Eye spasm is sometimes referred to as "pseudo-myopia." While "pseudo" refers to a temporary or false situation, prolonged near work may cause the temporary myopia to become permanent.[21]

How this happens is not clear. Other factors, such as poor lighting, glare, even stress have also been implicated in the development of myopia or nearsightedness. But it is important to remember (and vision scientists will quickly point this out) that just because two events occur at the same time does not mean that one causes the other.[22]

Does Scholastic Competition Effect Eyesight?

I asked my son to take the SAT exam when he was 12 years old. If he scored well he would be offered a summer enrichment program at Johns Hopkins University!

I'll never forget the expression on his face when he came out of the exam. He was dazed.

"Why did you make me take that test?"

My reply:

"Nicholas, in order to do well in life you have to go to a good college; in order to get into a good college you have to do well on the SAT exams; in order to do well on the SAT's you have to practice and prepare."

He just stared at me.

"My head hurts!"

At that moment, I truly understood how academic competition had affected my behavior toward my children. We can place a great deal of pressure on our children to keep up academically. It starts early with tutors, music lessons, summer enrichment programs, and continues on with SAT prep courses, private schools, etc.

As parents, it's understandable that we want our children to have a competitive edge, but this drive to excel can take its toll. Increased near work limits the range of focus to 12 to 16 inches and limits physical activity as well. Life is about balance.

Does Wearing Eyeglasses Make My Child's Eyesight Worse?

While the short answer to that question is, "No," it's not always that simple.

Eye doctors have wrestled with this topic for years! It was once thought that wearing eyeglasses that fully corrected vision and provided children with perfectly clear, 20/20 vision encouraged eyesight to worsen and ultimately

> My daughter, Kelly, had her initial pair of glasses when she was 7 years old. At that time her eyes were -2.00. Her vision rapidly got worse. By age 11, both of her eyes were already -6.00, with no signs of stopping. As parents, my wife and I were both very anxious.
>
> —Hong

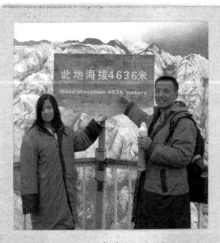

Kelly (B) with her dad, Hong

此地海拔4636米

Here elevation 4636 meters

require stronger and stronger eyeglasses. It was believed that if the child looked at near objects through the fully corrected distance lenses it would require the eyes to work harder and they would get worse. Because of this, many eye doctors would under correct a child's vision in the distance by prescribing eyeglasses that were weaker than needed.

Other eye doctors disagreed and felt a child's vision should be corrected fully so he had the best chance at good vision. I used to recommend that children wear eyeglasses for watching TV and looking at the board in the classroom, but take them off when they did near activities. While that was great in theory, it rarely worked in reality since the eyeglasses would get lost; or the child would never take them off; or worse yet, never put them on!

Some optometrists thought a great solution to this problem was to prescribe bifocal eyeglasses. These allowed children to see out of the top of the lenses for distance viewing and look through the clear lower portion for reading. Once again, in theory this should have worked. But in reality, it rarely helped slow down the progression of myopia in our children.[23]

However, it's not that simple, especially for children who spend a great deal of time performing near work. Be sure to question any doctor who believes there is only one approach to prescribing eyeglasses for children.

My Story Could be Your Story

When parents hear the news that their child is nearsighted, it can create a sense of bewilderment, feelings of guilt and lots of questions. I know; I lived it. When a parent hears the news that their child has myopia, we now know that there are many factors that contribute to its development. Genetics, culture, increased near activities and lack of outdoor activities all may play a role.

My story may be similar to yours. The narrative of a young child being diagnosed with myopia is written countless times every day in eye care practices around the world.

When you are told your child has myopia, it may seem like hard news to handle. But, the good news is that there are a lot of resources out there to help you and many options available to help your child.

I'm here to help because I'm not only a parent just like you,
I'm an eye doctor, too.

Part I Highlights

- Genetics plays a large role in the development of myopia or nearsightedness, but it is not the only factor and may not be the most significant factor.

- The development of nearsightedness is also influenced by near work activity and the amount of time your child spends outdoors.

- Culture and environment will also play a role in the development of nearsightedness.

How We See

Barry M. Tannen, OD

Part II

In the United States…up to 1.6 million school-age children have vision problems.

I'm an eye doctor, a parent and also an optometric educator. For the majority of my professional career, I have taught optometric students that there is more to vision than 20/20 eyesight. There is a human being behind the eyes we examine; a concept that can be overlooked in our fast paced medical system. So when Dr. Despotidis asked me to educate parents on the role of eyesight in our children's lives, I embraced the challenge. My goal is to educate you without boring or overwhelming you. Here are some of the questions parents ask me daily:

"What is 20/20 vision?"
"What is the difference between farsightedness and nearsightedness?"

The eye is an amazing part of the body! Through the eye and the vision it provides, the world opens up before us. However, problems with vision can begin at any age and are even found in very young children. Early detection and treatment is essential to prevent these vision problems from getting worse as a child grows.

By the age of three, most experts agree that our children have the potential for adult-like vision. But in the United States, up to 1.6 million school-age children have vision problems. However, as few as 14% of American children receive an eye exam before entering first grade.[24]

What Are the Different Parts of the Eye and How Do They Work?

The eye is made up of several different parts that all work together to provide vision. To help you understand how vision works, it is important to understand various parts of the eye. Don't worry, we won't go through all of them, but let's take a look at the ones that play the largest role in vision. We've also added a glossary in the back of the book for your reference.

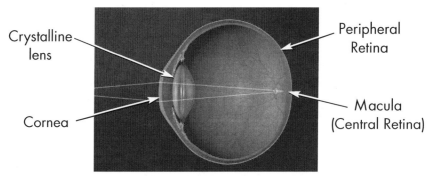

Crystalline lens

Peripheral Retina

Cornea

Macula (Central Retina)

The **cornea** is found on the very front of the eye and acts like a car windshield. It is transparent and allows light to pass right through it. Since it is curved, it bends the light rays when they enter so they focus on the correct spot on the back of the eye. The curve of the cornea plays a big role on where those light rays land (we'll discuss that more a little later on).

The **iris** is what gives our eyes color. When we talk about green eyes, blue eyes, brown eyes or hazel eyes, we are really describing the color of the iris. The iris is also partly responsible for regulating the amount of light permitted to enter the eye.

The iris is made up of muscles that make the ***pupil*** (the hole in the middle of the eye) either larger or smaller. When more light is needed, the pupil gets larger. When the light is too bright, the muscles in the iris will make the pupil smaller to restrict the light coming in.

The ***crystalline lens*** (or simply the lens) is a transparent structure inside the eye that focuses light rays onto the retina. While its role is to focus light (just like the cornea), it can actually provide various powers depending on how it is stretched by the muscles holding it (unlike the cornea). In our children, this ability to change focus (called ***accommodation***) is very strong. Unfortunately, if you're reading this with bifocals or reading glasses, the ability of your lens to change focus isn't quite as powerful. This normal change usually happens around the age of 40 and is called ***presbyopia***.

Positioned in the back of the eye is the ***retina***. This light sensitive lining of the eye receives the image of what is being viewed and sends it to the brain for interpretation. Vision doesn't actually take place in the eyes. Instead, it takes place in the brain.

When we look at an object at a distance, the object's image is focused on the back of the eye (the retina). When the image is focused clearly, it is focused on the central part of the retina called the macula. When everything lines up perfectly and the image is centered right where it is supposed to be, it is called ***emmetropia***. A person who is emmetropic has perfectly focused vision without the use of eyeglasses or contact lenses.

What is Nearsightedness?

We want the images to fall perfectly on the retina in the back of the eye, but they don't always do that. If the image falls *in front* of the retina instead of on the retina, the person is nearsighted (also called myopia). That means that vision close up is good, but far away it is blurry. The greater the amount of nearsightedness, the blurrier or fuzzier things become at a distance.

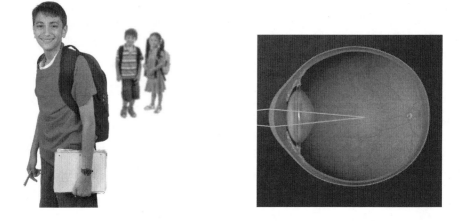

Myopia or nearsightedness happens when the eye is slightly longer than usual, so the light rays come to a focus closer to the front of the eye. Why does this happen? There is no one clear answer to this question, but the good news is that there are things that can be done to provide good vision to nearsighted people and actually halt its progression.

People who are nearsighted need either eyeglass lenses or contact lenses that will refocus the light rays further back in the eye so they fall on the retina.

What is Farsightedness?

Farsightedness, as you might expect, is the opposite of nearsightedness. Instead of the light rays falling in front of the retina, they fall

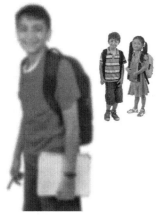

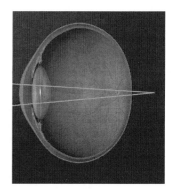

behind the retina. (Okay, not actually behind the retina, but they would if they could.) In these cases, the eye is too short, rather than too long. With farsightedness (also called hyperopia), objects that are far away are clearer than objects up close.

Eyeglass lenses and contact lenses can help to refocus the light rays closer to the front of the eye and provide good vision for people with farsightedness.

So, What is Astigmatism?

Astigmatism sounds serious, but it is really a very common vision condition! As a matter of fact, most of our patients have some degree of astigmatism.

Astigmatism occurs when the shape of the cornea (front surface of the eye) isn't perfectly round. Therefore you can envision the shape of the cornea to be more oblong (like a football) than spherical (like a baseball). This means that light rays don't focus in one spot on the retina, but focus in two different spots instead. This makes vision blurry at every distance. If astigmatism, especially in high degrees, is not corrected it will cause eyestrain and fatigue.

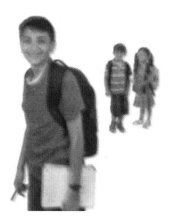

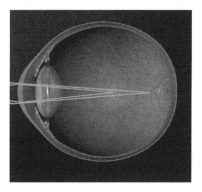

What is 20/20 Eyesight?

When I say "normal vision" what is the first thing that pops into your head? If you're like most people, the first thing that comes to mind is 20/20 eyesight. But what does 20/20 eyesight really mean?

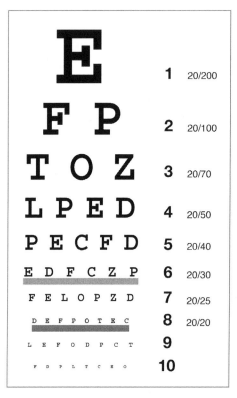

Around 1862, a man named Herman Snellen devised a testing system to measure people's eyesight. He had individuals stand 20 feet away from a chart and through experimentation he discovered the smallest sized letter that most people with good eyesight could see clearly. He called this a size 20 letter and the vision was recorded as 20/20. At the time it was considered the only test needed to determine ideal vision. Now, over 150 years later, we have made quantum leaps in our knowledge of the vision system.

Being able to see 20/20 on the eye chart tells us how well we can see to drive. It can tell us how well our children can see the board at the front of the class. It tells us if we can see a newspaper or a computer screen.

But there are many things "20/20 eyesight" will never tell us. It will never tell us if you or your child:

- sees clearly all day long
- can focus back and forth between the board at the front of the room and the book on the desk

- sees single images rather than double images
- can read without getting a headache
- can follow words on a page without losing the place
- can read without wanting to fall asleep
- has healthy eyes

And all of these things are important! It is critical that the health of the eye, as well as the vision, is carefully evaluated every time an eye exam is performed. This makes yearly eye health examinations so critical. While the focus of this book has been correcting children's vision to 20/20 at distance, I have to emphasize that 20/20 is only part of total eyesight!

How Did the Visual System Develop?

Let's talk about vision 500 years ago. Why would that be important? Understanding how our visual system evolved can help us to understand the demands we place on our vision today. What did we need vision for 500 years ago? People then needed vision to hunt for food and to keep from becoming food! Both of these tasks required good vision…at a distance! Our visual system evolved to allow us to see clearly far away. But how things have changed!

- 500 years ago the first printing press was invented, making reading materials more accessible
- The Industrial Age increased the need for near work 150 years ago when factories sprang up
- Compulsory education was instituted in America about 100 years ago
- And over the past 30 years, the advent of personal and business computers has increasingly brought our world closer and closer

Today, near vision tasks make up the majority of our workday, yet our visual system evolved for distance tasks. This creates an inherent mismatch between what our eyes are developed to do and what our eyes need to do, resulting in strain. So it's no wonder that a major complaint of computer users is eyestrain. Because of the widespread stress created in today's society, behavioral optometrists have developed extensive examination techniques and treatment recommendations based on the Nearpoint Visual Stress Theory.[25, 26]

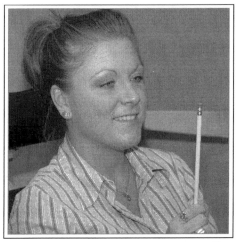

Let me show you what nearpoint visual stress is for yourself. Take the index finger of your right hand and hold it out in front of you at the same level as your nose. Focus on the tip of your finger and slowly start bringing it toward your nose. Keep moving it closer until you feel some discomfort or stress in your eyes or your forehead. Just keep your finger at this position. This is your nearpoint visual stress point and it is different for everyone. Some people's nearpoint visual stress point is very close to their nose, while others can be one or even two feet from their nose.

Imagine a typical child spending hours each day doing schoolwork, working on computers, playing computer games. These are all done at near distances. How can this child respond to this nearpoint visual stress?

One way they adapt is to develop physical changes in their eyes to handle difficult situations. They need to see near? They give up distance vision. This is a child who:

- holds things very near
- squints when he looks up from reading books
- has difficulty copying from the board at school
- eventually becomes myopic or nearsighted

Of course there are genetic factors at work as well, but the amount of near work performed is becoming more and more of a factor as we research the cause of nearsightedness.

Having your child examined by an eye doctor who performs a thorough nearpoint vision analysis is important for the healthy development of your child's visual system. Remember, a healthy eye means more than 20/20 vision.

───── My Story Could be Your Story ─────

I have two children, Rachael and Noah. Understanding the nature of how our children's eyesight develops, and with a little luck, they've reached adulthood without the need for eyeglasses.

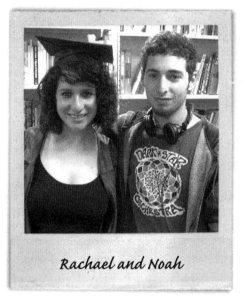

Rachael and Noah

Part II Highlights

- Early detection and treatment of vision problems is essential to prevent them from getting worse as a child grows.

- Near vision tasks make up the majority of most people's days, yet our visual system evolved for distance tasks. This creates a mismatch between what our eyes are developed to do and what our eyes need to do every day.

- Healthy vision means more than 20/20 eyesight!

How Do I Help My Child?

Ivan Lee, OD

—————— Part III ——————

*By the year 2020 myopia will affect
2.5 billion people worldwide.*

It's my training. If there is a problem, I find a solution. If a patient has an eye infection, I prescribe medicine. If a patient is nearsighted, I prescribe eyeglasses or contact lenses. My training made me feel well prepared for the challenges I'd face as an eye doctor. Unfortunately, there wasn't such clear cut training for the challenges I'd face as a parent.

I have two children, Tristan and Gillian. My son is a bookworm. Even though he is just starting to read, he always has his head in a book. As a toddler, he loved books and that love grew when he became a preschooler. When I performed his latest eye exam, I found that Tristan was showing signs of early myopia or nearsightedness.

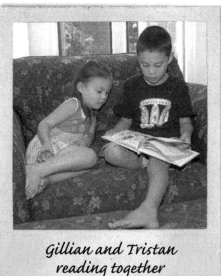

*Gillian and Tristan
reading together*

He's only 5 years old!

I was dismayed. I am engaged in research involving myopia. I have special training in new techniques to handle and control nearsightedness. I routinely prescribe eyeglasses for children who need them and update the prescription if there is a problem. I've been in practice for over a decade and during this time I rarely gave much thought to myopia and why it occurred in some children and not in others. That is, until my role as a father collided with my role as an optometrist.

Drs. Tannen and Despotidis showed me how to incorporate a holistic approach to the care of patients, especially children. Instead of simply asking a child, "Which is better, one or two?" we have more of a functional approach to vision examinations and correction. We don't simply ask what image or letter is clearer on the eye chart; we ask how the child is using their eyes.

> Does your daughter play sports?
>
> How often does your son play video games?
>
> How long does he work on the computer?
>
> Is she an avid reader?
>
> How many hours does she read each day?
>
> What kind of extracurricular activities does
> your child participate in?

It is this functional approach that helps us not only diagnose a problem but also uncover several layers of a treatment plan and address a patient's potential underlying problems.

So what am I going to do, as a doctor and as a parent, to halt or slow the progression of Tristan's nearsightedness? Since my story may be similar to your story, let me share with you the many options that are available to my young son and to your child as well.

Why Do Children's Eyes Get More Nearsighted?

Peripheral Retina

Nearsighted

Central Retina

Peripheral Retina

A   B

As Dr. Tannen discussed, an eye that doesn't need help with vision correction focuses light rays on the back of the eye on the area called the retina (A). When an eye is too long, light is focused in front of the retina (B). When conventional corrections are used, like traditional eyeglasses and contact lenses, the light rays are focused solely on the very central part of the retina (C).

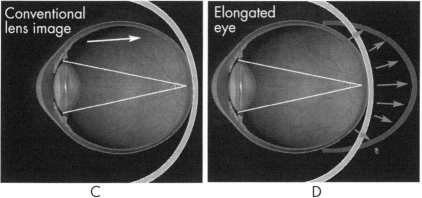

Conventional lens image

Elongated eye

C   D

Conventional lenses leave the peripheral retina unfocused.

Unfocused peripheral cells move toward image elongating the eye.

Animal studies have shown that myopia (especially high degrees of myopia) can be caused when the peripheral or outer areas of the retina don't get a clear image and light rays there remain unfocused.[27-30] The cells in the unfocused area begin to move toward the image away from the retina and ultimately make the eye longer (D). If this is the case in humans, it is an unfortunate pattern that keeps repeating itself when conventional eyeglasses or contacts are prescribed. Glasses focus light only on the central portion of the retina, beginning this cycle of myopia. The same tools that doctors prescribe for nearsighted patients do nothing to control myopia from getting worse.[31, 32]

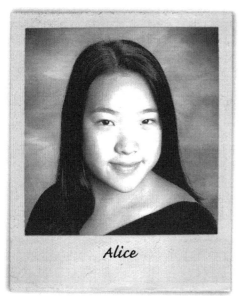

Alice

Excessive close work, like reading or playing video games, is another reason a child's eyes may get more nearsighted. Some research supports the theory that when a child is focusing hard for reading or other near tasks, the contraction of the eye muscles may cause the overall length of the eye to increase. This increase in length will cause the child's eyes to become more nearsighted.[33-35]

Prolonged near work may also tire the eye muscles. This fatigue causes the light rays to focus behind the retina. Unfocused areas on the retina lead to migration or movement of the cells and unfortunately an eye that gets longer and more nearsighted.[27, 29, 30]

"I am a certified bookworm. When I was young, I would read nonstop, never imagining it would have its downside. In 6th grade I got my first pair of glasses, but even glasses didn't stop my vision from getting worse.

—Alice

How Can I Help My Child?

The only factor I could actively control for my son, Tristan, was his environment. Let's go through the good vision habits I instituted in my household. Remember, sometimes the simplest changes can make the biggest difference.

Hold Reading Material 14 Inches Away

The closer a child holds a book, the harder the eyes have to focus to maintain a clear image. Encourage your child to keep reading material, the computer monitor, handheld games or any near work at least fourteen inches away.

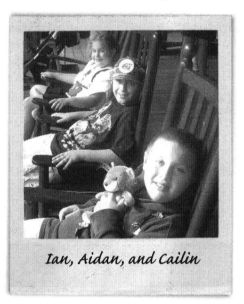

Ian, Aidan, and Cailin

If your child continues to move his head closer and closer to the material, this may be a sign of a vision problem. There are many vision issues that would cause a child to move a book closer to his eyes. If you notice this behavior with your child, I'd encourage you and your child to visit an eye doctor who emphasizes a behavioral approach

> From the time they began reading on their own, all three of my children would move closer and closer to the book when reading. On the advice of our family eye doctor, I started teaching them from a very young age to use better posture while reading. It took constant reminding at first, but it has now become a healthy habit.
> —Jennifer (mom)

to eye examinations. The College of Optometrists in Vision Development (COVD) certifies professional competency in this approach. You can visit www.COVD.org for more information and to find an eye doctor in your area.

Rest Every 30 Minutes

If a child reads a book, works on a computer or plays video games for hours at a time, it can potentially cause vision problems. I encourage children to stop a near task every 30 minutes. Get up and move! Having children break from the near activity and walk around gives vision a break, too. I know, this is easier said than done. Children can be so engrossed in reading, playing a video game or working on the computer that it can take considerable effort to even get their attention. I recommend setting a timer to act as an alarm. If it's in the same room as the child but on the other side, the simple task of checking how much time remains will get them to change to a distance focus.

Play!

Encourage your child to play and move around. The more time they spend playing video games, watching TV and reading, the less time they spend doing things that require distance vision. As we've seen in the previous chapter, spending too much time on near tasks can contribute to nearsightedness.[3]

Play Outside!

We can take this one step further. Encourage your child to play outside. The human body produces Vitamin D when exposed to sunlight. Vitamin D is important in maintaining calcium metabolism and insulin secretion, among many other interactions that keep us healthy.[36] Without Vitamin D and calcium, the eye's structure (collagen) could be weakened and the eye might have an increased chance of getting longer.

This increases the chance of myopia occurring.[37, 38]

The role of sunlight in the development of the eyes is currently a topic of particular interest. In a study of Australian school children a key finding was that the lowest myopia rates in 12-year-olds were associated with high outdoor activity, independent of the level of near work activity. The research showed that it was the sunlight, rather than simply playing in a particular sport that was the critical factor; playing indoors in a gym had no positive effect on controlling myopia.[20] There may be factors other than sunlight that can explain this result. For example, when playing outdoors children focus at further distances and the use of artificial lighting indoors may have negative effects on vision. Even with these other factors, sunlight may play an important role in regulating our children's eyesight.

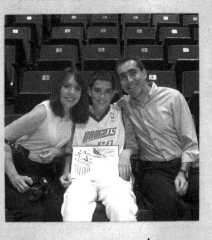

Teresa, Gregory and Dr. D

"When Gregory was younger we encouraged him to play outside, a task we thought he'd enjoy! But to our dismay, he'd sometimes prefer to work on his computer, read or play video games. We noticed several kids in our neighborhood didn't play outside as often as we used to as children."

—Dr. D.

Kids today are so busy with indoor activities that it leaves less time at the end of the day for good old-fashioned outdoor fun. Yet, it's this very important outdoor time and sunlight that are so important to the healthy development of our children's eyes.

Use Good Posture While Reading

I feel proper posture is critical to maintaining good vision. Proper posture allows our children to maintain an appropriate equal distance from their reading material. This element of equal distance can sometimes be overlooked, but I feel it's very important. When I examine

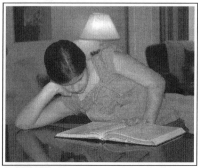

Don't Lean

children who have very different prescriptions between their two eyes, I'll often discover that they've developed a habit of reading or writing with their head tilted. While it's hard to say if the head tilt occurs because of the difference in the two eyes, or the head tilt caused the difference in prescriptions, it's wise to have your child practice good posture and proper reading distance.

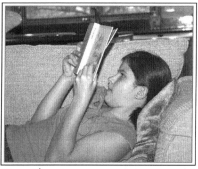

Too Close

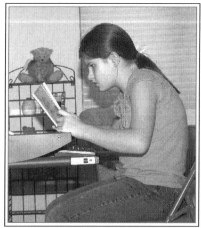

Poor Posture

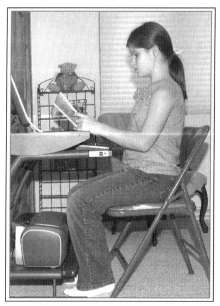

Good Posture
Back straight, book tilted, feet on floor and good distance from book

Here are some tips to avoid eye strain:

- Make sure both feet touch the floor. If your child's feet can't reach the floor, have him sit in a smaller chair or place something beneath his feet.

- The reading material should be tilted back at a 20-degree angle.

- Watch for rolled shoulders! Make sure the child is sitting upright in the chair.

- Place reading material directly in front, not off to the side. This is especially important when viewing a computer monitor.

- Ask that your child not read in bed. This is because the distance from the material to the eyes isn't controlled. When children read in bed, their posture may be distorted.

- For the same reasons mentioned above, make sure your child doesn't tilt his head or rest it on the desk when he reads or does near work. If your child continues to tilt his head when he is reading, even if you've corrected him many times, schedule a visit with the eye doctor.

- Light the space. I recommend an adjustable 60-watt incandescent lamp and avoid any source of glare on the reading material.

Do Carrots Help My Child See Better?

This is a question I get from a number of parents. The answer is, "Not really…" We know how nutrition may help prevent diseases such as macular degeneration and cataracts.[39-41] But very little is written on the effect our children's nutrition has on their vision development.

In his book, "The Myopia Manual," Klaus Schmid provides a wealth of information on myopia, its possible causes and suggestions for prevention.[42] Schmid is quick to point out that just because there is a commonality between nutrition and vision development, it does not mean there is a cause and effect relationship.

As Schmid points out, "Generally more rigorous schooling and higher advanced technology are going hand-in-hand with a change in nutrition and increased mental stress." The number of refined and processed foods our children consume is far greater than when we were younger. There is simply more of it available and in our conven-

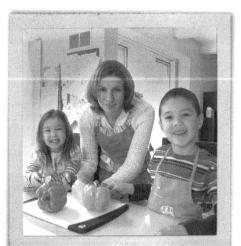

My wife, Kim having fun with our children

> " I stress the importance of a proper diet. A typical meal includes fresh fruits, vegetables, lean meats and only whole grain carbohydrates. All our dairy items are non-fat or low fat. We found healthy alternatives for most foods. For example, our kids love pancakes on Saturday mornings; I serve whole wheat pancakes with skim milk. "
>
> —Kim

ience-driven society, the call is more alluring.[43] What this specifically has to do with the increased number of myopic children in my exam chair is yet to be seen.

As with other aspects of our children's lives, there should be a healthy balance in their diet. My recommendation is to strive for a diet low in sugar and other simple carbohydrates like white bread, white pasta and white potatoes. Minimize salt intake and saturated fats found in foods like French fries, butter and other fast foods. Encourage a diet high in fruits and vegetables.

Doesn't this sound like the common sense recommendations you hear all the time? They are. And they are the same ones that people should follow regardless of their age! The U.S. Department of Agriculture (USDA) and U.S. Department of Health and Human Services (HHS) updated their nutrition guideline for Americans.[44] Their recommendations? Eat less, make wise food choices and, of course, be active!

Preliminary research has shown that diet may have an impact on the stability of the connective tissue of the eye. When the connective tissue is weak, it is easier for the eye to get longer and become myopic.[45, 46]

Foods rich in refined carbohydrates and sugar increase blood sugar and insulin levels. Elevation of these levels is a strong stimulator of tissue growth; including tissue in the eye, which may allow the eye to elongate.

A conclusion can be drawn that the development of myopia may actually be increased by a high sugar and processed food diet.[47, 48]

Here are recommendations I offer my patients regarding their diet:

- One daily multi-vitamin
- Limit sugar in the diet

- Limit simple sugars from white foods like
  white rice, white bread, white pasta and potatoes
- Limit saturated fats by reducing junk food
- Eat plenty of vegetables and fruits
- Encourage a diet rich in "good fats" like omega-3
  found in nuts and fish (assuming there are no allergies)

As with all changes in your child's daily regimen, make sure to consult with the pediatrician.

More than likely, as with most other things, the development of myopia in children occurs because of a combination of events: genetics, increased near work, less outdoor activities, reading environment as well as the food our children eat.

I've Heard that Some Doctors Prescribe Eye Drops for Children ——— With Nearsightedness. Is that True? ———

Wouldn't it be great if something as simple as an eye drop or gel could prevent or cure nearsightedness? In some countries, including the United States, eye doctors prescribe eye drops for children with myopia. But these drops don't prevent, nor do they cure, nearsightedness. Instead, the eye drop, called atropine, slows down the elongation process of the eye, therefore slowing down the progression of myopia.[49-51]

Atropine is similar to the drops used by eye doctors to dilate your pupils during routine eye examinations, but is much stronger.

It affects our children's eyesight by preventing their eyes from focusing up close. Children who are given atropine drops or gel cream need to wear reading glasses to help them see near objects. Initially, it was thought that temporarily stopping the eyes from focusing on near objects was how the drops slowed nearsightedness. Now, vision scientists believe that atropine and other similar drops send a chemical signal to the eye telling it to stop the growth that creates myopia.[52] Regardless of the mechanism, atropine works in slowing down the progression of nearsightedness. Atropine therapy is effective for a period of one to two years and, after that point, the eye is less responsive to the drug and its effectiveness stops.

Despite atropine's effectiveness, we don't prescribe it in our office. Why? The reason for us is simple; atropine has too many negative side effects. Atropine dilates the pupil, creating a great deal of light sensitivity. Children taking atropine have trouble reading (because their focusing ability has decreased with the drops) and seeing outdoors (because they are sensitive to light). Atropine drops can even make our children feel tired and sluggish, making it hard to simply be a kid!

So although atropine has tremendous potential, in its current formulation

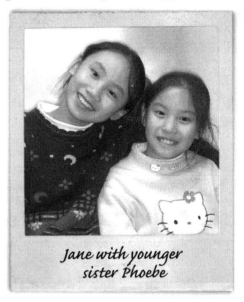

Jane with younger sister Phoebe

> Jane was 7 years old when she first required eyeglasses. Her vision continued to deteriorate, so when her eye doctor recommended eye drops in an effort to slow down her eyesight from getting worse we were optimistic. Unfortunately, they made her eyes very sensitive during the day and her vision continued to change. Her prescription increased so fast and eyeglasses bothered Jane, so we took a friend's recommendation and tried corneal reshaping lenses.
>
> —Roger (dad)

its side effects outweigh its benefits for me to use it with my son. Some eye doctors disagree.[53] If your child's eye doctor recommends this therapy for your child, I'd recommend asking them to prescribe the drops for you for a week to better understand the risks and benefits.

—— How Should Eyeglasses be Prescribed? ——

Dr. Despotidis mentioned earlier some eye doctors were taught to prescribe less power or under correct a child's eyeglasses. This strategy was supposed to reduce the amount of focusing our children needed when they were reading. A prescription for distance work (like seeing the board in school) can sometimes be too powerful for reading and this leads to excessive strain on the eyes. Also, some believe that a child should never wear a full prescription because she will "get used to" the full prescription and will eventually become more nearsighted at a rapid pace.

Recent studies suggest that under correcting a child's prescription does not slow down the progression of myopia. As a matter of fact, two studies showed it may even make it worse![31, 54] When I prescribe eyeglasses for a child, I prescribe the full power that will allow my patient to see as clearly as possible at distance and near. Sometimes this requires the use of separate reading glasses or even bifocals to maintain clarity of near vision.

Bifocals? Will They Work For My Child?

Using bifocals or progressives (lenses that provide a gradual shift of power from distance to near) for children has been a controversial subject. With bifocal and progressive eyeglasses, the distance correction is provided in the top portion of the lens and the near correction is provided in the bottom.

Bifocals or progressive lenses can help some children maintain clear vision, especially if they have trouble keeping letters in focus when they are reading. Other children may have a tendency to cross

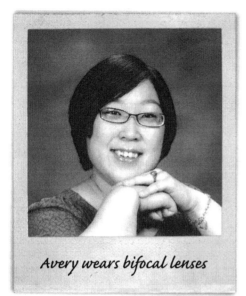

Avery wears bifocal lenses

> When the doctor recommended bifocals for our daughter, Avery, I was shocked, if not saddened. He explained that bifocals would help her focus properly while reading. Now, several years later we're happy we followed his recommendation as Avery continues to wear them and loves to read.
>
> —Tirrell (mom)

their eyes while they are reading (esophoria), which can also be helped by wearing bifocals.

While bifocals seem to help children who have problems focusing or over crossing when they read, the reality is that the majority of children do not have these issues.[55] Your child's eye doctor will determine if bifocals are the best option to help your child see well up close, prevent eyestrain and ultimately prevent the eyes from becoming more nearsighted.

I've Heard LASIK Will Correct Nearsightedness. Will it Work For My Child?

LASIK stands for laser assisted in situ keratomileusis, the medical term used to describe laser eye surgery used to correct myopia. While this is a successful treatment for myopia, it is an elective surgery. The FDA guidelines state that a patient must be at least 18 years of age before they undergo LASIK. There are eye care practitioners (I'm one of them), who prefer to wait even longer. I recommend young adults wait until they are finished with college (and all of that intense near work) before considering LASIK.

LASIK is a very safe and accurate procedure when performed by a skilled and experienced surgeon. However, it's not free of problems. Although most surgical outcomes are ideal and most patients are very happy, there is a chance of experiencing permanent, devastating visual symptoms after treatment. Although very rare, I've examined patients who have experienced vision loss, severe dry eye, as well as glare and halos around lights after LASIK surgery. These and other issues experienced by LASIK patients can be found detailed in the FDA website, www.FDA.gov.[59] LASIK works by changing the front surface of the eye (the cornea) by removing very small amounts of tissue. This tissue, once removed, cannot be replaced.

> I've had very poor vision since childhood and have worn glasses and contacts most of my life until I had LASIK. Every time my daughters would have an eye exam I would secretly pray neither had inherited my vision. Unfortunately, my younger daughter Julia was the unlucky one. One day I asked her to read something for me and she couldn't, confirming my fear; her eyes were becoming as bad as mine.
>
> —Toni

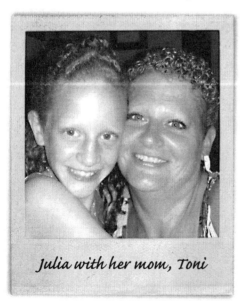

Julia with her mom, Toni

The results of LASIK, good or bad, are permanent!

I believe LASIK is best left for adults over the age of 25. Although we treat all of our patients on an individual basis, we know most young adults continue to experience changes in their vision as they continue through school and beyond. Before we consider LASIK for any patient, we make certain that the patient's vision has not changed in at least a year. If your teenage son or daughter brings up LASIK as an option to get rid of their eyeglasses or contact lenses, assure them that it can still be discussed as an option when they complete their schooling.

How Old Does My Child Have to be to Wear Contact Lenses?

It's a question I hear a lot and the answer may surprise you. There is no age requirement for wearing contact lenses. Even infants with some medical conditions wear them.

But even for non-medical reasons, research has shown that children as young as eight years old can be fit with contact lenses.[60] In our office, we fit children as young as five when the situation is right. Even though contact lenses are a safe option, as with most things, there is always a risk. In the case of contact lenses, the introduction of bacteria and potential infections always makes us weigh those risks against the benefits before we fit children.

Another question commonly asked by parents is whether or not wearing contact lenses will help to keep their child's vision from getting worse. Soft contact lenses will do nothing to impact the progression of myopia. If a child is going to get more nearsighted, they will whether soft contact lenses are worn or not.[61]

Gas permeable contact lenses (made from a more rigid material than soft lenses) have a *very slight* ability to control myopia. Unfortunately, the amount is *not* enough to warrant prescribing rigid gas permeable contact lenses as a means to slow down myopia.[62, 63]

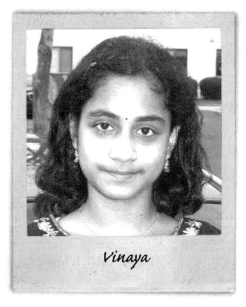

Vinaya

We still remember that distressful day in our life when our daughter, Vinaya, who was 10 at the time, came home from school holding her broken glasses. Today, Vinaya wears corneal reshaping lenses and is a happy child. She got rid of her glasses and her confidence is up!
—Srinivas & Sireesha (parents)

However, there is one important reason to consider contact lenses for your children, even if they don't necessarily slow down the deterioration of their vision (myopia); self-esteem! Currently there is a study designed to determine if wearing eyeglasses affects our children's self-esteem.[64] Although the results are not yet available, clinically I've seen some children's personalities blossom after they replaced their eyeglasses with contact lenses! It's interesting because this does not happen with all children; but when a change in self-esteem occurs, it's immediately evident to the parents and everyone around them. If your child shows an interest in contact lenses, discuss this with the eye doctor. But wait for your child to approach you. Contact lenses are not for everyone, so let your son or daughter guide you.

Is There Anything That Will Stop Myopia?

Myopia is a leading cause of vision loss and it's estimated that by the year 2020, myopia will affect 2.5 billion people worldwide.[65] It is going to be an epidemic in many regions of the world. It's not uncommon for children wearing eyeglasses or contact lenses to have their eyesight deteriorate yearly. There is nothing that will stop myopia from occurring, but fortunately recent research indicates that there may actually be a way that the progression of myopia can be slowed down. Researchers have found that by wearing specially-designed gas permeable lenses overnight, called corneal reshaping lenses, a dramatic difference can be made in a child's vision.

And we've witnessed this in our office![69]

While many eye doctors aren't aware of this research and don't offer this type of treatment, the results of

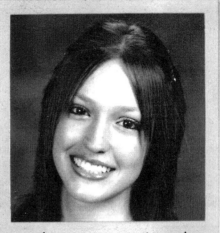

Elyse never experienced wearing eyeglasses

"At 9 years old, my daughter Elyse started to recognize her declining eyesight. When she could barely see the biggest "E" on the eye chart, I knew we had a big decision to make; corneal reshaping or glasses. Corneal reshaping was something I never heard of. I wanted to be sure my daughter received the best product and care. After all, it was her vision we were dealing with.

—Janice (mom)

these studies and our own clinical experience has definitely changed the treatment of nearsightedness in our practice.

In our next section Dr. Despotidis will explain what corneal re-shaping is and how it works.

My Story Could be Your Story

My dilemma with Tristan's emerging myopia and the prospect of my daughter, Gillian, some day needing eyeglasses may be a similar concern of yours. Hopefully, by reading this chapter you can better understand some of the reasons your child has been diagnosed with myopia and why it continues to progress.

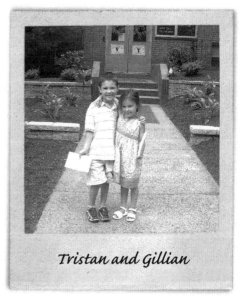

Tristan and Gillian

Your next step is to consider the recommendations outlined in this chapter. While they may be small, they are significant steps that you can take to positively impact your child's vision.

Part III Highlights

We've listed the three main reasons, other than genetics, that contribute to the development of myopia or nearsightedness and our recommendations to help your child below:

- Physical pressure placed on the eyes by reading and other near tasks
    - Hold images 14 inches away
    - Rest every 30 minutes when doing near work
    - Play ... outside!
    - Use good posture when reading or doing near tasks
    - Use good lighting and avoid glare

- Nutrition
    - Limit simple sugars and saturated fats in the diet
    - Eat plenty of fruit and vegetables
    - Encourage a diet rich in good fats like Omega-3

- The clarity of the image received by the retina at the back of the brain
    - Make certain your child has the best possible correction for their vision problems

Is Corneal Reshaping Right for My Child?

Nicholas Despotidis, OD

———— Part IV ————

Neither son remembers wearing glasses.

I fit my son, Nicholas, with corneal shaping lenses when he was in the fourth grade. While there was a lot of contemplation surrounding the decision, the fact that Nicholas despised wearing eyeglasses made it a lot easier! Another factor was that his eyesight had progressively gotten worse since he started wearing eyeglasses in the second grade. I knew what I had to do.

When I was in optometry school, orthokeratology (that's the technical term used for corneal reshaping) was viewed very skeptically. But this changed in 1992 when several improvements in contact lens materials were made. These new materials allowed significantly more oxygen to pass through the lens, making it safer to sleep with them in overnight. Computers also played a big part in the evolution and acceptance of corneal reshaping. Advances in computer programs allowed the eye doctor to monitor how well the treatment was working and make necessary changes to create a predictable and safe correction of a patient's myopia.

⸺ How Does Corneal Reshaping Work? ⸺

Corneal reshaping technology uses a carefully designed rigid oxygen permeable contact lens that gently changes the shape of the front of the eye, called the cornea, while you sleep. The lenses are uniquely designed for every child and are often different between one eye and the other. Interesting, huh? But how does this improve myopia or nearsightedness?

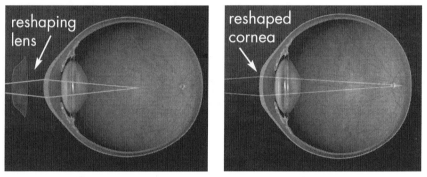

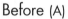

Before (A)   After (B)

When a person is nearsighted, it is because the eye is too long. This causes images to focus in front of the retina instead of on the retina (A). Corneal reshaping lenses flatten the front part of the eye and allow the image to focus further back onto the retina (B). That's a good thing since it is the retina that is responsible for receiving the images, converting them into electrical impulses and then sending them to the brain where they are "seen."

A child will apply these contact lenses in the evening before bedtime. As the child sleeps, the corneal reshaping lens correctly molds the cornea to the shape needed to properly focus light on the retina. When the child wakes, the lenses are removed. The best news is that because the outer layer of the eye has been reshaped during the night (kind of like braces on teeth), your child can see well during the day—without eyeglasses or contact lenses!

Corneal reshaping is one of the terms used for this new, emerging technology. Other resources may refer to it as orthokeratology, OK Lens, Ortho-k, Corneal Refractive Therapy (CRT®), or Vision Shaping Therapy (VST™). In our practice, we use the term Gentle Vision Shaping System (GVSS™).

I've Never Heard of Corneal Reshaping. Is it New?

Corneal reshaping is a relatively new area of eye care and I'll be the first to admit that there is still some controversy surrounding its use. Because of this, it shouldn't come as a surprise that some eye doctors may not be supportive of this option for your child. Some of the uncertainty on their part may be based on false reports they've heard or bad

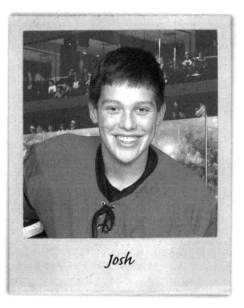

Josh

> Our eye doctor suggested Josh would be a great candidate for corneal reshaping lenses. I was quite skeptical…two friends who are eye doctors strongly urged us against their use. Now, as I look back 2 years later, I can honestly say that Josh has been liberated from the "threat" of having to wear corrective eyewear during the day.
> —Carine (mom)

experiences they've had with the old technology. It can also be because they simply haven't researched the treatment thoroughly enough. If you encounter an eye doctor who is less than supportive, I would recommend you get a second opinion from an eye doctor who is familiar with this treatment option. Then, decide what is best for your child.

There are several websites that can help you locate eye doctors who

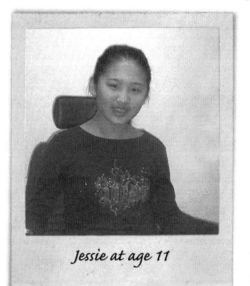

Jessie at age 11

show interest in corneal reshaping technology. While these websites are great resources to start your search, they don't take the place of a face to face consultation. Unfortunately, being listed on one of these websites does not insure proper proficiency with corneal reshaping lenses, nor can they take into account the comfort level needed to make this a successful treatment.

"I inquired about corneal reshaping from a doctor in China. He promptly told me if Jessie was his daughter he would never allow her to wear these lenses! When Jessie's eyesight continued to deteriorate, I visited another eye doctor but his advice was similar. A third doctor recommended corneal reshaping; I was confused and frustrated. Fast forward 2 years after proceeding…Jessie's vision is stable and she does not wear eyeglasses during the day. I feel my search for the right treatment for my daughter was rewarded."

—Jie (mom)

The Orthokeratology Academy of America (OAA) administers voluntary corneal reshaping certification of eye doctors through an extensive written and practical examination. While this organization is still in its infancy at the time of this writing, it is a good resource to help parents and patients locate a doctor in their area. Visit them at www.okglobal.org.

These other websites may also be helpful for your research:

    www.Bausch.com
    www.Ortho-k.net
    www.ParagonCRT.com

It is important to find an eye doctor who sincerely cares about your child. During the first consultation visit, a physician's commitment to your child's well-being should be evident. If you and your child are comfortable with the office, doctor, staff, explanations, and treatment parameters, then that is the practice for you. Follow your intuition.

Can Any Eye Doctor Fit Corneal Reshaping Lenses?

A different question may be, "Why don't all eye doctors offer corneal reshaping lenses to their patients?" The reality is that most eye doctors do not perform corneal reshaping! Okay, I know what you're thinking. "Why not?!"

Bottom line, it takes more time and effort to fit corneal reshaping lenses than regular contact lenses. It involves a more in-depth knowledge of the fitting of rigid contact lens materials, and it requires specialized equipment that not all eye doctors have in their offices. There is also additional certification needed to be able to fit corneal reshaping lenses.

But time, knowledge and equipment aren't the only reasons many eye doctors don't take on corneal reshaping in their offices. Becoming proficient at corneal reshaping, explaining the process and treatment to parents and patients all takes time; and it's not time that every practitioner has or wants to devote. (When was the last time a medical professional devoted twenty minutes or more explaining a medical option to you and your child?) Most parents have never heard about corneal reshaping technology, a key inspiration for writing this book!

In addition to time, patience is often required to work with children. While the technical aspects are the same as they are for adults, children often come to the exam room more frightened, nervous or fearful than their adult counterparts. Unfortunately, many eye doctors get used to running from

> My older son Frank started wearing corneal reshaping lenses, but he wasn't able to see well during the day. After struggling for 2 years, we changed doctors. Within a few weeks his vision improved significantly! Now, my younger son, James, wears them. Both boys enjoy sports without having to worry about glasses or contact lenses. I am a physician and highly recommend parents consider corneal reshaping for their children who need glasses.
>
> —Shufang

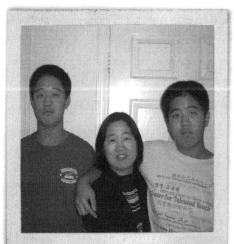

Shufang with sons, Frank and James

exam room to exam room, quickly (but efficiently!) diagnosing patients, prescribing treatments and then hustling off to see the next patient. It's go, Go, GO! It's truly an investment in knowledge, equipment, time and patience. Bottom line, if the eye doctor doesn't enjoy what he's doing, the treatment won't be successful.

How Do We Get Started?

The first step is to determine if your child is nearsighted and requires eyeglasses. An eye doctor will determine an accurate eyeglass prescription and confirm that your child's eyes are healthy. The next step is to locate an eye doctor who is experienced with corneal reshaping (we'll help you with that at the end of this book) and schedule a consultation.

What Happens During the Consultation?

Every individual office will, of course, handle the consultation differently. But, I can give you an idea of what would happen by describing a typical consultation in our office.

The first step is to measure the shape of the front surface of your child's eye (remember, that's the cornea). The instrument used is called a corneal topographer. It measures the curvature of the front of the eye in thousands of different points, helping the eye doctor to precisely design a corneal reshaping lens that will safely and effectively correct the patient's vision. Amazing!

After the initial lens design has been determined, a diagnostic lens is placed on the child's eye to determine how well the lenses are tolerated. Corneal reshaping lenses are made from a rigid material, yet unlike older contact lens materials, are extremely oxygen permeable. Children will feel the lenses when they move their eyes, especially when they blink, but it's important to remember that this sensation is only temporary.

Even though the child won't feel the lenses while sleeping, there can still be some apprehension on the part of the child or the parents. Sometimes, when I sit across from children, I can see the fear and worry etched on their small face.

"Will it hurt?"
"Will I be able to put them in?"
"What if I can't get them out?"
"What if they get lost in my eyes?!"

This is the part of the consultation that requires patience--from the parents, the children and the doctors! I've seen children as young as five do well with the lenses and teens as old as sixteen refuse to let us near their eyes. Giving the child something to distract their attention can make the time pass more quickly for everyone involved (we use snacks!). Once the child has had a chance to relax with the lenses on, about 15 minutes or so, the fit of the lenses and vision are evaluated.

It would seem obvious that your goal as a parent is to find an experienced eye doctor who specializes in corneal reshaping, who addresses the technical element that is necessary to provide your child with a successful result. But, it is also your goal as a parent to find an eye doctor with a personality and office that makes your child feel comfortable and at ease. You and your child will spend a lot of time at the specialist's office and those are visits you don't want to dread. Doing your homework up front and taking the time to find the right eye doctor for your child's vision treatment will pay dividends for years to come.

The consultation is a critical step in the fitting process. It provides valuable information about the ultimate fit of the corneal reshaping lenses, helps to assess a child's reaction to wearing the lenses as well as gives you the opportunity to evaluate the atmosphere, making certain it is the right one for you and your child.

Is Every Child a Candidate?

There are so many corneal reshaping success stories (just take a look at the back of the book!). But, unfortunately, there are a few times when it doesn't work. In our office, if we place diagnostic lenses on the child's eyes and the anxiety level doesn't lessen, or it even increases, we ask the parents to bring their child back when they are a little older. It doesn't make any sense to create anxiety for the child or the family when it can be a more effective (and pleasurable!) experience by waiting until the child is truly ready.

Another reason a child may not be a candidate is if the eye doctor can't achieve a good fit even after trying multiple diagnostic lenses. In this situation, the doctor may discourage you from going any further with the treatment. This can happen when the shape of the eye and the prescription won't allow effective correction of your child's vision.

However, the good news is as technology advances, more and more FDA approved corneal reshaping lenses become available. And not only does the arsenal of corneal reshaping lenses and designs increase, but eye doctors are becoming more experienced with fitting this technology. Every year, the likelihood of your child being a corneal reshaping candidate improves.

How Does My Child Learn to Handle the Contact Lenses?

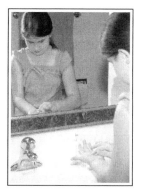

After the initial evaluation, the next appointment typically involves a class for your child to learn how to apply and remove the corneal reshaping lenses on their own. In our office, in order to "graduate," your child must be able to apply and remove the lenses at least three times in each eye. Children will also learn how to clean and care for their corneal reshaping lenses and will need to demonstrate the techniques before the corneal reshaping lenses are released to them. While some children will require their parent's assistance for the first few weeks, it is important that children learn how to handle and care for their corneal reshaping lenses on their own, no matter how young they are!

We realize that this can be a time of stress for the child and for the

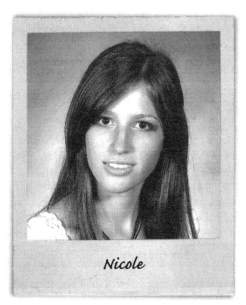

Nicole

parents. It is a lot of responsibility for a young child, and a new experience for the family (especially if the parents don't wear contact lenses themselves!). And it doesn't come easily to all children. My younger son, Gregory, needed to take the class five times before he graduated! Even though he was only 7 years old at the time, it was vital that he was comfortable with the

> We were all very concerned that Nicole would not be a candidate for corneal reshaping because of her strong aversion to anything in her eyes. The doctor was so patient and explained that this process takes getting used to. As a parent, I was concerned that we would spend all this money and she wouldn't be able to get through the initial discomfort…it's been a few years now and Nicole can put the lenses in her eyes in minutes and refuses to sleep without them! I still have trouble believing that she did it.
>
> —Rhonda (mom)

application, removal and care process on his own. And the good news is that he was able to do it (finally!).

Perhaps it's because of my personal experience as a father and an eye doctor that our office has developed multiple techniques that help make the "class" pleasant, yet effective as possible. For instance, prior to the class we provide the family with a DVD that outlines the basic techniques we'll cover when they return to learn to apply and remove the lenses on their own. This gives the family some valuable insight well before the big day.

This initial appointment is full of information and instructions and regardless of how carefully we present the information or how closely the family listens, questions are bound to come up. Communication is key! To offer assurance and guidance and address any questions or concerns that may have come up, our office calls patients during that all important first week. We continue to correspond with all of our corneal reshaping patients through email or telephone to address questions and concerns (yes, email, if you can't beat them join them!). We're just a click away!

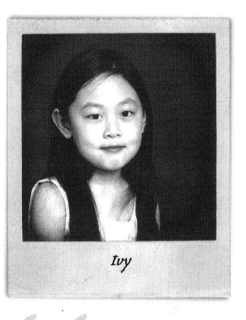

Ivy

Dear Dr. D,

Guess what? I did it!!!

It took me less than 2 minutes to put my lenses in last night and 5 minutes to take them out this morning. What type of prize should I get for this excellent job?

Thank you for your support.

Love,
Ivy

To help the process along, we suggest parents develop a reward system for their child. Some children are just not motivated, they simply don't mind wearing eyeglasses or are too young to understand or care about their progressively deteriorating vision. So we develop leverage! For instance, when children initially learn how to handle their corneal reshaping lenses, they get a reward of their choice from their parents (within reason of course!). After a week and then a month of successful wear, they receive another reward. Getting children started on the right foot will help to put them on a path to lifetime success. In this case, "bribery" works. It's a time-tested technique that's helped apprehensive children through those initial few days.

Patience is so important! Even young children who may be terrified of having anything placed on their eyes can become extremely capable of handling their lenses. But the support of parents is crucial!

What do you do if the parent is determined and excited about wearing the lenses, but the child lacks the fine motor skills to place them on his eyes? This is common among our younger patients, as they are too young to understand the purpose of wearing corneal reshaping lenses and can be understandably frightened. In these isolated instances we ask the parent to help! If the parents are comfortable, they can help the child apply the corneal reshaping lenses at night. But, it is important to only do this until the child matures enough to do it alone. Becoming successful with this type of technology takes total commitment from both the parent and the child! After one to three months, the lenses become more comfortable, the vision has been perfected and at that time the child can begin to apply the lenses on his own.

My Kid is a Kid!
How Will He Keep the Lenses Clean?

Parents are naturally concerned about their children properly caring for the corneal reshaping lenses. We look at the mess in our children's rooms or the dirt on their hands and can't imagine that these young people can safely care for these tiny medical devices! But remember, sketchy hygiene isn't limited to children! We all know adults who are messier than our children and the manufacturers of care products have taken that into consideration when making the solutions effective in spite of the possibility of human error.

Good hygiene is obviously critical for success when wearing corneal reshaping lenses. The good news is that procedures are kept simple, so it is not difficult for children (and even most adults!) to follow instructions accurately and consistently, making problems rare.

How Long Does the Treatment Take?

Once the customized corneal reshaping lenses are ordered for your child, we anticipate between 6 and 10 visits to the office the first year. Children are able to see clearly and go to school eyeglass free after just a few nights of sleeping in their lenses and glasses are rarely needed after their first week of wear! Afterwards, several visits are needed to "perfect" the vision and lens fit. About 90% of the children we see in our office have stable vision within the first year.

Follow-up visits are critical to the successful fitting of corneal reshaping lenses. At every visit, your child's vision and eye health will be evaluated. Corneal topography is used to monitor how effectively the treatment is working. This computerized equipment allows us to determine where the lenses were resting on the eye while the child sleeps—even after the lenses are removed! It can even help us determine whether the lenses are fit too tightly or too loosely and allow us to make adjustments to the fit. Corneal topography is a critical evaluation that should be performed during follow-ups and is a necessary part of the process. If the eye doctor you have chosen does not perform corneal topography, they will not be able to accurately fit or follow your child's progress.

How well your child is cleaning and caring for the corneal reshaping lenses is another area that should be evaluated at each follow-up visit. Proper care of the corneal reshaping lenses is such a vital part of success that it needs to be monitored constantly. When the wear and care regimen is new, there may be instructions and directions that are unclear, so getting the child started on the right track is critical. But, even after the routine has become established, a shortcut may slip in or an important detail may be missed, so it is important to continuously monitor the process. Not only will the fit of the lenses be checked at every visit, but the cleanliness of the lenses and the case will be evaluated as well.

The number and timing of follow-up visits will vary from doctor to doctor and will also depend on how well your child's eyes are responding to the treatment. Most practices (ours included) will see the patients regularly during

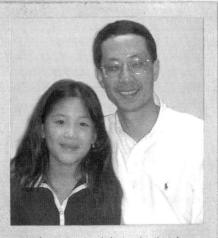

Stephanie and her dad, Sheng

I was at the checkup and the result was perfect for Stephanie! After so many rounds of hard work and patience, we finally saw the great results we hoped for. We really appreciate your effort and are very grateful to you for the great work, patience and wonderful treatment you have given to my daughter. Many thanks from the bottom of my heart!

—Sheng

the first year during which time most of the changes occur, the bulk of the learning and the most challenging days take place.

What happens if the child's vision isn't as good as expected? If your child isn't seeing well throughout the day, adjustments will be made to the shape of the corneal reshaping lenses and new lenses will be ordered. We treat all our patients as if they were our own children. This means if we determine that a new set of corneal reshaping lenses will improve the fit or vision, we order them! This is an important distinction to make when selecting a doctor to work with your child. In our office, the number of changes we make are not limited. We continue to make changes during the first year until an optimal balance of fit and vision is achieved, even if it goes beyond the initial fitting period. Period! But, this isn't the case with all practices, so it is important to understand what philosophy is followed by the eye doctor that you choose to treat your child.

Which Corneal Reshaping Lens is Best?

The good news is there are a number of corneal reshaping lens designs available, since one lens design can't fit all children safely and effectively. The "best" lens design is the one that works for your child. Your eye doctor may be comfortable with several different designs and will choose the one they feel is best for your child's particular situation. Sometimes the first choice does not work as expected, so it helps to have more than one lens design to use.

My two sons wear lens designs from two different manufacturers. It didn't start out that way, but through the fitting process, it is how it ended up. The result; they are happy and I am happy! But, it also emphasizes why it's important to find an eye doctor that is experienced with fitting more than one lens design. If not, some potentially successful patients may be considered failures. Not all corneal reshaping lenses fit everyone.

How Much Does the
⎯⎯⎯ Corneal Reshaping Treatment Cost? ⎯⎯⎯

Now, that's a good question! Of course, I can't answer that question for everyone fitting corneal reshaping lenses, but I can offer some insight into how the fees are determined. The corneal reshaping process is often bundled into a package program helping to save you and the eye doctor from unexpected fees. A typical program will include the consultation, the fitting of the corneal reshaping lenses, follow-up visits, as well as additional lenses needed to improve the fit or vision. Some packages will include other options, such as a spare pair of lenses once the fitting is complete. We include an extra pair of lenses, understanding that lens loss and breakage are common during the first year of treatment. Each pair of corneal reshaping lenses lasts about one year, at which time they need to be replaced.

Program fees can range from hundreds to thousands of dollars. A wide range exists because of the many variables that can be included in the package. The program fees will also depend on the amount of time the eye doctor thinks they will need to spend with your child. When comparing and evaluating different corneal reshaping providers, it is important to remember to compare apples to apples and make sure an orange hasn't slipped in there! For example, if one eye doctor charges a fee for a package that includes the consultation, fitting, follow-up visits, but limited or no lens exchanges for a fit modification, it may not be the best "deal" when compared to another eye doctor who includes any and all changes made. It is important to fully understand not only what is involved with the program, but what is included in the fees as well.

It is obvious that you should never select a doctor based on fees alone. The time invested in finding a doctor who interacts well with your child pays great dividends for years to come and not only leads to a more successful outcome, but a happier child.

How Much Does Insurance Cover?

Unfortunately, since corneal reshaping is not considered a medical necessity, most medical and eyeglass plans do not cover the cost of the treatment, visits, or lenses. But, many offices will offer various payment plan options to assist parents and families, which may include discounts for paying in full or interest free financing so payments can span several months.

When Does My Child Stop Wearing Corneal Reshaping Lenses?

Children wear corneal reshaping lenses nightly—forever. If they stop, over the next few days their vision will slowly return back to baseline. Corneal reshaping treatment is not permanent. And that is its benefit! Unlike laser eye surgery (LASIK), corneal reshaping technology does not permanently alter the eye's structure.

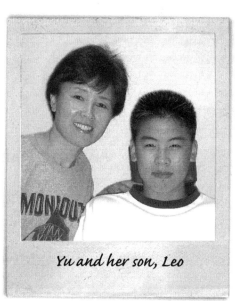

Yu and her son, Leo

Wearing corneal reshaping lenses every night is not any less convenient than brushing our teeth. As a matter of fact the majority of our patients who start wearing corneal reshaping lenses as children continue to wear them into their adulthood!

> As a veteran of corneal reshaping for almost eight years, wearing these lenses every night has become as routine as brushing my teeth.
>
> —Leo

And we encourage this, at least through college. And as we discussed earlier, throughout their academic years is when our children's eyesight has a tendency to worsen. Rarely do any of our corneal reshaping patients return to regular contact lenses or eyeglasses. We also have a large number of adults who wear corneal reshaping lenses (some over the age of 60!) simply because many adults dislike wearing eyeglasses or contact lenses and are either not candidates or don't want to have surgery that will permanently alter their eyes.

The lenses must be slept with nightly for 6-8 hours to ensure excellent vision throughout the waking hours. What happens if a corneal reshaping wearer doesn't wear the lenses for a night? After all, they are kids! I'll admit that my children skip nights when they are not feeling well, they fall asleep in the car or they just don't get around to applying the lenses. If they skip a night, their vision the following morning is not as clear. How unclear depends on the original eyeglass prescription. If two nights are skipped, the vision is even blurrier. We discourage skipping nights because it can easily become a habit (like skipping brushing your teeth). So, to have the best results, kids have to wear their corneal reshaping lenses nightly to maintain clear vision during the day.

This All Sounds Great, But is Corneal Reshaping Safe?

These are our children we're talking about! This makes safety the most important issue. However, as with everything, even with the safest procedure, product, treatment or medication, there is a risk. There is no way to eliminate all of the risk, but there are ways to reduce the probability of the risk.

Any contact lens placed on a child's eyes will introduce risk that isn't present when a contact lens isn't worn. But, the probability of a problem occurring has been reduced with today's newest materials that allow more oxygen and improved lens designs that reduce interaction with the eye. Since the risk remains, it is important that the fitting and follow-up, wearing and caring are taken very seriously and directions are followed.

Eye infections are perhaps the most feared side effect of wearing any type of contact lenses. When we place any lens on our eye, soft or rigid, disposable or corneal reshaping, we introduce germs. While there are certainly reports of children acquiring infections, some even very serious, most of these infections occur outside of the United States.[70] There are also studies that have demonstrated the safety of corneal reshaping lenses for children.[71]

Still, as an eye doctor who fits corneal reshaping lenses for children, as well as a father with two sons wearing them, the reports of risks concerned me. So, as a result, I became involved in a task force whose job was to investigate this very topic. The group included ophthalmologists, vision scientists, optometrists and educators throughout the United States and abroad.[70] After the investigation concluded, it was determined that there was not enough data to determine if corneal reshaping lenses expose our children to a greater risk than ordinary contact lenses. The task force also developed a series of recommendations that can minimize the risk to our children who wear all types of contact lenses.

All of our patients, no matter how young, agree to the following directives:

- I agree to wash my hands before applying or removing my lenses.
- I agree to clean my lenses each time I remove them.
- I agree not to rinse my contact lenses in water from the sink.
- I agree to tell my parents if my lenses irritate my eyes.
- I agree to immediately tell my parents if my eye appears red or painful.

Children are carefully taught to care for their corneal reshaping lenses and are monitored at every visit to make certain they are following our instructions. With our children's safety first in our minds, diligence is the last thing we'll give up!

Thousands of children currently wear corneal reshaping lenses, including my own two sons. I strongly believe the benefit of clear vision during the day and the possibility of stabilizing my sons' nearsightedness far outweighs the possible risk of wearing lenses.

So, are corneal reshaping lenses safe? Yes! Do they introduce risk to our children's eyes? Yes, but realistically the risks are rare and steps can be taken to avoid them. And let's not forget that there are risks associated with nearsightedness as well. As a child's eye becomes more nearsighted, it gets longer. This stretches the back lining of the eye (the retina) and puts the child at a higher risk for conditions such as a retinal detachment. High degrees of nearsightedness also increase the risk of developing diseases like glaucoma and cataracts.[6-11]

This is the main reason I sit down with parents considering corneal reshaping for their children and discuss with them all the risks, benefits, realities and myths. Together, we have a discussion about whether corneal reshaping is right for their child. It is the same discussion you should have with the eye doctor you have chosen.

My Story Could be Your Story

Corneal reshaping was the right choice for my children. I was hesitant about fitting my youngest son, Gregory, at the young age of seven. Yet, I also wanted to be proactive and attempt to slow down his nearsightedness. Fast forward more than ten years and I am certain we made the right decision since his eyesight has not changed. Neither he nor his older brother, Nicholas, remembers when they wore eyeglasses! They've grown into young, confident adults who have played sports, marched in the school band, swam like fish, went to dances and now drive; all without the hassle of eyeglasses. The hard work and determination early on has certainly paid off. To my kids, I'm just their dad…goofy at times, but willing to do whatever it takes to give them the best opportunity for a great future.

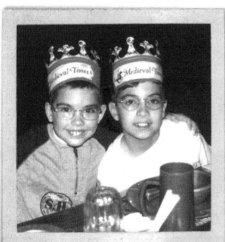

Gregory and Nicholas
Ages 7 and 9

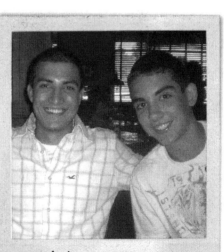

Nicholas & Gregory never
remember wearing glasses

Part IV Highlights

- Corneal reshaping technology involves wearing a rigid, oxygen permeable lens that gently reshapes the front of the eye while the child sleeps.

- Corneal reshaping treatment is not permanent. And that is its benefit! Unlike laser eye surgery, corneal reshaping technology does not alter the eye's structure permanently.

- Preliminary research and clinical experience has found children who wear corneal reshaping lenses do not experience prescription changes as rapidly as children wearing eyeglasses or contact lenses.

- While an important goal is to find an experienced eye doctor who can effectively and efficiently fit corneal reshaping lenses, it is also important to find an eye doctor with a personality and office that makes your child feel comfortable and at ease.

- The key word throughout the corneal reshaping process is patience and it is important from the part of the patient, the parents and the eye doctor. With patience and support, even young children can be very successful.

Author Biographies

Nicholas Despotidis, OD

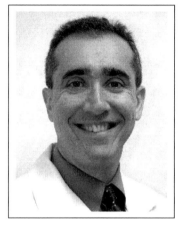

Dr. Despotidis and his wife Teresa are the parents of two sons, Nicholas and Gregory. It was his children's need for eyeglasses at very young ages that sparked his passion for corneal reshaping and drove him to become a pioneer in its use among children and young adults. "Dr. D" (as his patients fondly refer to him) has been practicing optometry for over 20 years and strives to bring a heightened level of compassion to every individual in his care.

Dr. Despotidis graduated with honors from The State College of Optometry in New York and later completed a residency in Vision Therapy/Pediatric Vision. He is a Fellow in the American Academy of Optometry and is a Board Certified Fellow in Vision Therapy with the College of Optometrists in Vision Development. He has published papers in optometric journals and is a frequent lecturer. He is co-founder of EyeCare Professionals, P.C., in Hamilton Square, New Jersey.

Dr. Despotidis is a 4th degree black belt in Tae Kwon Do Karate and co-founder of Martial Arts With Hearts (MAWH) a philanthropic organization started with his instructors Bryan Klein and Michael Crocco. MAWH has raised hundreds of thousands of dollars for children afflicted with autism, birth defects, cystic fibrosis and cancer.

Ivan Lee, OD

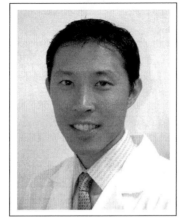

Dr. Lee and his wife Kim have two children, Tristan and Gillian. Dr. Lee's family originated from Taiwan and he is very much attuned to the higher incidence of nearsightedness (myopia) in patients who share his heritage. As a Fellow in the American Academy of Ortho-keratology, Dr. Lee is a leading expert in the field of corneal reshaping and has been featured in the PBS series, "Asian America," discussing the incidence of myopia in Asian students.

Dr. Lee attended Rutgers College for his undergraduate studies and obtained his Doctorate of Optometry at Nova Southeastern University College of Optometry in 1997. He completed an internship at Bascom Palmer Eye Institute in Miami, Florida, and his residency in Ocular Disease at the Wilkes-Barre Veterans Administration Medical Center in Wilkes-Barre, Pennsylvania. He entered private practice with EyeCare Professionals, P.C., in 2001.

Barry Tannen, OD

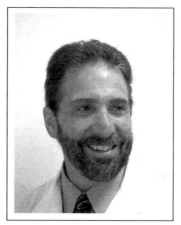

An optometric physician for over 25 years, Dr. Tannen's career has been devoted to the diagnosis and treatment of children with vision problems that impact academic performance. Dr. Tannen is a passionate doctor who cares deeply about the children he examines and treats. He and his wife Sandi have two children, Rachael and Noah.

Dr. Tannen graduated with clinical honors from the Pennsylvania College of Optometry. Dr. Tannen is an Associate Clinical Professor of Optometry at the SUNY/State College of Optometry in New York where he teaches vision therapy and is also the Director of the Eye Movement and Biofeedback Clinic.

Dr. Tannen is a Fellow in the College of Optometrists in Vision Development and the American Academy of Optometry. In 2002, he was the recipient of the New Jersey Society of Optometric Physician's Scientific Achievement Award. Dr. Tannen lectures nationally and internationally on learning related vision disorders, strabismus, amblyopia, and vision therapy. He has co-authored a clinical textbook as well as published numerous papers. He served as an officer in the United States Public Health Service for three years before cofounding EyeCare Professionals, P.C., with Dr. Despotidis.

Clearing Up Eye Terms

Nicholas Despotidis, OD

—————— Appendix A ——————

Atropine – Atropine is a medication applied directly to the eye that temporarily dilates the eye and paralyzes the ability to see up close. Check out Part Three where the use of atropine in children with progressive myopia is discussed in more detail.

Accommodation – Accommodation is the term used to describe the ability of the eye to focus on objects up close. Children normally have a much greater ability to focus on near objects than adults. This ability weakens as a person ages and that's why adults need *bifocals* or reading glasses after the age of forty.

Astigmatism – One term used to describe a condition of the eye is astigmatism. When light rays don't come to a single focus, but instead focus in two different spots (making our vision blurry at all distances), eyeglasses and contact lenses are needed that have two different powers Even though it might sound scary, astigmatism is a very common eye condition!

Behavioral Optometry – "Functional optometry" is another name for behavioral optometry. This is an expanded area of optometry that uses a holistic approach in the treatment of vision. Optometrists who pursue this type of practice are interested in how vision impacts children's daily lives. They undertake postdoctoral certification in the College of Optometrists in Vision Development *(COVD)*.

Bifocal – Bifocals are eyeglasses or contact lenses that have two separate powers in different segments; one for distance vision and the other for near vision. In most cases, the top segment provides distance vision and the bottom segment provides near. We've highlighted the use of bifocals for children in Part Three.

Cataract – A cataract is a clouding of the *crystalline lens* found inside the eye and you may be surprised to discover it's a normal part of aging. Everyone eventually develops cataracts, often in their sixties. However, cataracts have been reported at earlier ages among people with high degrees of *myopia (nearsightedness)*.

Cornea – The clear outer portion of the eye is called the cornea. This is the part of the eye that is first responsible for bending light rays when they enter the optical system. The cornea is permanently altered during *LASIK* eye surgery. The cornea is also the part of the eye that contact lenses rest on and is temporarily reshaped with *corneal reshaping* contact lenses.

Corneal Reshaping – Corneal reshaping is also referred to as *orthokeratology*, ortho-k, Corneal Refractive Therapy (*CRT®*) and Vision Shaping Treatment (*VST™*). (This is why we wrote this book; it's so confusing!) Corneal reshaping describes the use of specially designed contact lenses used only at night to correct *nearsightedness (myopia)* during the daytime. The technique is completely reversible, unlike *LASIK*, which makes it ideal for children and others who do not want to wear eyeglasses or undergo surgery. In addition, preliminary studies indicate children who wear corneal reshaping lenses do not progress in *myopia* as rapidly as kids wearing daytime contact lenses or eyeglasses.

Corneal Topography – A computer driven instrument that accurately measures the very front surface of the eye (*cornea*) in order to more properly fit contact lenses and *corneal reshaping* contact lenses is called a corneal topographer. Corneal topography is a must for the proper fitting and follow-up of corneal reshaping contact lenses.

COVD – COVD stands for College of Optometrists in Vision Development. Fellows of the College (FCOVD) have certified their competency in this area and often refer to themselves as *behavioral or functional optometrists*. For more information visit www.COVD.org.

Crystalline Lens – The lens inside the eye that focuses light rays is called the crystalline lens. Remember *accommodation* (it's at the beginning of this section)? The crystalline lens is the structure of the eye that is responsible for changing focus so we can see objects both up close and far away, or accommodate. When there is a lack of transparency or cloudiness in the crystalline lens it is called a **cataract**.

CRT® – CRT or Corneal Refractive Therapy is the acronym used to describe the corneal reshaping lens designed by Paragon Vision Sciences, a contact lens material manufacturer. In 2002, CRT was the first *corneal reshaping* lens to receive FDA approval. For more information visit Paragon's website at www.ParagonCRT.com.

Esophoria – As our children read, we assume their eyes are working together as a team, allowing them to scan across the page efficiently. This is not always the case. When our children's eyes have a tendency to over converge or point inward, eye doctors refer to this eye teaming problem as esophoria. There are different degrees of esophoria, which can be addressed with *bifocals* or *vision therapy*.

FAAO – We often notice letters providing our doctor's credentials, but what do they stand for? Fellow of the American Academy of Optometry (FAAO) is a postdoctoral recognition for optometrists and other health professionals who voluntarily demonstrate the highest standards of professional competence after undergoing rigorous testing and case presentations.

Farsightedness – When a person's eyes can focus more clearly on objects far away than objects up close, it is called farsightedness or *hyperopia*.

FOAA – The Orthokeratology Academy of America (OAA) is a newly formed organization committed to educating the general public and eye doctors about *corneal reshaping*. Practitioners who submit patient cases involving corneal reshaping and pass written and oral examinations are certified as fellows (FOAA) within the academy. For more information visit www.Okglobal.org.

Fovea – The fovea is located in the center of the *macula*, a region of the *retina*. The fovea is responsible for sharp central vision and is where the clearest, sharpest vision takes place.

Glaucoma – Glaucoma is a disease where high pressure within the eye causes damage to the optic nerve, the nerve leading from the eye to the brain. Glaucoma is treatable with a daily regimen of eye drops; but if left untreated it will eventually cause blindness. Glaucoma is painless and does not have visual symptoms in its early stages, so it must be detected by an eye doctor. People with high degrees of *myopia (nearsightedness)* are known to have a higher incidence of glaucoma than the general population. Other characteristics that increase the risk of developing glaucoma are a positive family history, age, African American or Asian heritage, diabetes and high blood pressure.

Hyperopia – Hyperopia is another term for *farsightedness*. When a person can focus on objects far away and has trouble seeing objects up close, they are hyperopic or farsighted.

Iris – The colored part of the eye is the iris. When you refer to someone's eye color, you are really referring to the iris color. Even more importantly than providing a physical trait, the iris contains muscles that allow the *pupil* to get larger and allow in more light or get smaller and restrict light.

LASIK – Laser assisted in situ keratomileusis (LASIK) is one form of laser eye surgery. LASIK corrects *nearsightedness* by permanently changing the outer layer of the eye called the *cornea*. LASIK is currently approved for patients older than 18, although many eye doctors recommend waiting until the completion of academic studies before considering it. A starting place for research into this procedure is the FDA website www.fda.gov.

Macula – When visual acuity is discussed, we are really talking about the sharpness of focus on the back of the *retina* called the macula region. Within the macula is the *fovea*, which is responsible for clear, central vision.

Macular Degeneration – Macular degeneration is the deterioration of the *macula*, the area of the *retina* that is responsible for central vision. Degeneration of the *macula* often leads to vision loss. The likelihood of macular degeneration increases with age and is also associated with high degrees of *myopia*.

Myopia – The vision condition in which objects are clear up close but blurry far away is called myopia or *nearsightedness*. Myopia can be corrected with eyeglasses, contact lenses and *corneal reshaping*.

Nearsightedness – The common term for *myopia* is nearsightedness. When a person has blurry vision at a distance but clear vision or sight at near, they are said to be nearsighted. A person may have nearsightedness in one or both eyes, with or without *astigmatism*.

Ophthalmologist – A medical doctor (MD) who specializes in treating diseases and disorders of the eye and performs eye surgeries, like *LASIK*, is an ophthalmologist. Ophthalmologists also prescribe eyeglasses and contact lenses. There are several subspecialists within ophthalmology, including pediatric ophthalmology.

Optician – An optician traditionally works along with *ophthalmologists* and *optometrists* by filling eyeglass prescriptions and fitting eyewear. Some opticians are also qualified to fit contact lenses.

Optometrist – Optometrists (OD) are a major provider of vision care. Optometrists perform eye examinations, diagnose and treat vision problems and eye diseases. Drs. Despotidis, Lee and Tannen are all optometrists.

Orthokeratology – The term used to describe the temporary improvement of *nearsightedness* with the use of specially fit contact lenses is called orthokeratology. The updated term used to describe this technique is *corneal reshaping*.

Pseudo-myopia – The transient shift toward *nearsightedness* occurring after continuous reading and other near work (did someone mention computers and video games…) is called pseudo-myopia. Pseudo-myopia is detected during a thorough eye examination and is treated with eyeglasses, *vision therapy,* good vision habits or a combination of the three. If left untreated, it can lead to permanent *nearsightedness (myopia)*.

Pupil – The entrance by which light and other images enter our eyes is called the pupil. It appears as a black hole surrounded by the colored *iris* right in the middle of the eye. The pupil changes size depending on the surrounding light. In bright light it gets smaller and in dim light it gets bigger.

Retina – In the back of the eye, where images are received, is the retina. This thin layer acts like a camera film capturing the picture of what we're looking at before sending it to the brain where the image is interpreted and our perception of the world is created.

Retinal Degeneration – As the eye grows and stretches with progressive *myopia* or *nearsightedness*, the likelihood increases that the back of the eye (*retina*) will degenerate or lose its integrity. This degeneration can cause vision loss.

Retinal Detachment – A retinal detachment describes the condition where the *retina* peels away from the inside of the eye. Retinal detachments are painless and may start very small, but spread quickly leading to loss of vision. When a person has a retinal detachment, they will notice an increase of floaters in their vision, flashes of light and may even notice a curtain or veil obstructing a portion of their vision. Because retinal detachments can lead to permanent vision loss, if you suspect you or someone you know has a retinal detachment, they should be seen by an eye doctor as soon as possible. Retinal detachments are more likely to occur in *nearsighted* people, especially those with higher degrees of *myopia*.

Sclera – The visible, white part of the eyes is the sclera. It is made of strong connective tissue and helps to maintain the shape of the eyes.

Vision Therapy – Vision therapy is also referred to as vision training and is a specialized area of optometry devoted to enhancing vision. (Dr. Tannen explains how good eyesight is more than simply 20/20 vision in Part Two.)   Vision therapy trains the entire visual system, which includes eyes, brain and body. The goal of vision therapy is to train the patient's brain to use the eyes to receive information efficiently, interpret the information properly and, of course, react to what they see. Vision therapy is primarily practiced by a select group of doctors referred to as ***Behavioral Optometrists***.

Visual Acuity – Visual acuity is the term most often used to describe the clarity of our vision. 20/20 vision refers to how clearly we see a standardized group of small black letters at a distance of 20 feet. The larger the denominator (the number on the bottom), the larger the letters needed for a person to see them. So a person who has 20/40 vision is not able to see letters as clearly on the eye chart as the person who has 20/20 vision. 20/20 vision is considered by many to be "perfect" vision, but it is only one measure of how well a person sees and only indicates what is seen at a distance. (Check out Part Two for more information!). *The metric equivalent to 20/20 vision is 6/6 vision where the distance is in meters rather than feet.*

VST™ – Vision Shaping Treatment refers to FDA-approved ***corneal reshaping*** lenses and designs offered by Bausch and Lomb. To check out more information or find a doctor in your area that fits VST lenses, visit www.Bausch.com.

How to Read an Eyeglass Prescription

	Sphere	Cylinder	Axis
Right Eye (OD)	-3.00	-1.00	180
Left Eye (OS)	-1.00	-2.00	180

The ***sphere*** component indicates the amount of ***myopia (nearsightedness)*** or ***hyperopia (farsightedness)*** present. When a negative (-) sign is in front of the number it is myopia. When a positive (+) sign is in front of the number it is hyperopia. The higher the sphere number, the greater the amount of myopia or hyperopia.

The ***cylinder*** component indicates the degree of ***astigmatism***. This number may be positive or negative; but in either case, the higher the number the greater the amount of astigmatism (or how irregularly the eye bends light). The cylinder component requires an ***axis*** to show how the astigmatism is lined up in the eye.

What is My Child's Vision?

We get asked the question almost daily. Some parents want to know their child's visual acuity. Is it 20/20 or 20/40? Others want to know their child's eyeglass prescription. Is it -1.00 or -3.00? As we've discussed before, the larger the numbers, the poorer the visual acuity.

A person with 20/400 visual acuity has poorer vision than a person with 20/40. A child with a prescription of -3.00 has poorer vision than a child with -1.00.

So, how are they related? The visual acuity (numbers like 20/20 and 20/40) tells us the size of the letters that can be seen at twenty feet. The prescription (numbers like -1.00 and -3.00) tells us what power needs to be in the eyeglass or contact lenses so that 20/20 vision can be achieved. The chart below gives a very rough relationship between visual acuity and prescription.

Acuity	Estimated Prescription
20/20	-0.25
20/30	-0.50
20/50	-1.00
20/100	-1.50
20/200	-2.00
20/400	-4.00

Example: If your child has 20/100 visual acuity, his eyeglasses will require approximately a -1.50 lens for him to see clearly at a distance.

Notes from Parents

Now it's time to hear from some of the many parents who have had their stories rewritten through the use of corneal reshaping contact lenses. Take a look at some of their experiences, written in their own words.

*"Every time my daughters had an eye exam,
I would secretly pray neither one of them
had inherited my poor vision."*

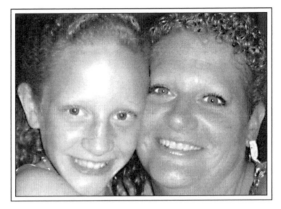

My name is Toni, a mother of two. I've had very poor vision since child-hood and have worn glasses and contacts most of my life until I had LASIK.

Every time my daughters would have an eye exam, I would secretly pray neither one of them had inherited my poor vision. Unfortunately, my younger daughter Julia was the unlucky one. One day I asked her to read something for me and she couldn't, confirming my fear; her eyes were becoming as bad as mine.

Our eye doctor gave us another alternative, corneal reshaping, I had never heard of it. It seemed like the perfect solution for us, Julia didn't have to wear glasses and I didn't have to worry about her wearing contacts every day. Yet I was skeptical. At 11 years old, I didn't think she would be able to handle contact lenses every day.

Julia is doing very well with this program and I feel extremely lucky that we were able to offer her this alternative to improve her vision. As a mom, the most important job I have is to make the right choices for my children; from the food they eat, to the schools they attend and the doctors they visit. I feel that I made the very best vision choice for my daughter.

Mom: Toni
Daughter: Julia

"Alyssa needed glasses starting in kindergarten."

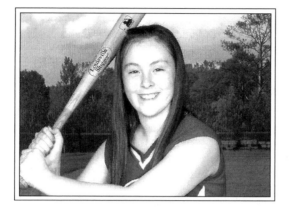

Alyssa needed glasses in kindergarten. The following year her prescription got significantly worse. At this time our doctor recommended something called corneal reshaping. I never heard of it, but was interested in any option that would prevent my daughter from having to deal with glasses or contacts during the day.

We started corneal reshaping when Alyssa was 6 years old. At first, it was a challenge putting in the lenses and especially removing them. Eventually Alyssa was able to take care of this process completely by herself, including cleaning the contacts each morning.

Now Alyssa is in the seventh grade! She never experienced wearing glasses or soft contact lenses. As someone who has been dependent on glasses and contacts, I know that Alyssa doesn't even realize how lucky she is! I really feel that having good vision every day has added to Alyssa's self confidence.

Alyssa has had a very positive experience with the corneal reshaping lenses. I tell all parents I meet whose children need glasses about them. The reaction I get is usually hesitation, but two of her cousins started wearing them this year.

Mom: Marykim
Daughter: Alyssa

*"I visited an eye doctor…their advice…
would not recommend this technology…
I didn't know which doctor to listen to."*

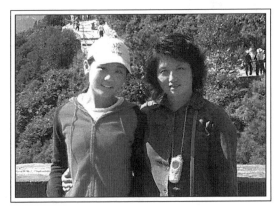

When the school nurse told me that my daughter Jessie was nearsighted, not only was my heart broken, I was also shocked! Both my husband and I have 20/20 vision. I never expected this could happen to my daughter.

I inquired about corneal reshaping from a doctor in China. He promptly told me if Jessie was his daughter he would never allow her to wear these lenses! When Jessie's eyesight continued to deteriorate, I visited another eye doctor but his advice was similar. A third doctor recommended corneal reshaping. I was confused and frustrated. I didn't know which doctor to listen to.

At age twelve, without much trouble, Jessie quickly learned how to wear the corneal reshaping lenses never needing my assistance. Fast forward two years later and she has not needed to wear eyeglasses or contact lenses during the day. My daughter is happy. I feel the year of searching for the right treatment has been rewarded. I would certainly recommend to other parents to consider this technology for their children if they wear eyeglasses.

Mom: Jei
Daughter: Jessie

*"I drove over one hour each way
to obtain this treatment."*

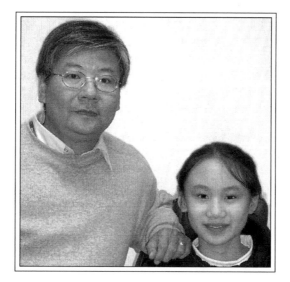

My daughter, Jane, was 7 years old when she first required eyeglasses. We were very saddened. Her vision continued to deteriorate, so when her eye doctor recommended eye drops in an effort to slow down her eyesight from getting worse we were optimistic. Unfortunately, the eye drops were not a good option for Jane. They made her eyes very sensitive during the day and her vision continued to change. Her prescription increased so fast and eyeglasses bothered Jane, so we took a friend's recommendation and tried corneal reshaping lenses. I drove over one hour each way to obtain this treatment. It was not easy. It required several trips to the eye doctor in the beginning, but we're very pleased with the outcome. That was over 6 years ago! Jane has not worn eyeglasses since and her prescription is stable.

Dad: Roger
Daughter: Jane

*"I am extremely nearsighted and
I require thick eyeglasses."*

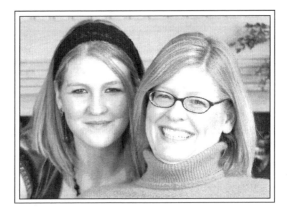

Similar to what had happened to me in my childhood, Emily had been wearing glasses since second or third grade, and her vision continued to deteriorate with each check-up. I am extremely nearsighted and I require thick eyeglasses. My husband and I did not want Emily's vision to grow worse throughout her teen and early adult years.

We decided to try corneal reshaping lenses and at first Emily had a difficult time adjusting to the rigid lenses. She felt they were uncomfortable and irritated her eyes. With great support and encouragement Emily persevered and adjusted to wearing the lenses in a couple of weeks. We are so glad that she did!

Emily is now in high school and an A student who takes her schoolwork very seriously. Her lenses have allowed her to maintain her vision, and to not worry about lenses during school or after school activities.

We are grateful that we learned about corneal reshaping while Emily was still fairly young and her vision loss had not progressed too far. I recommend the lenses to other parents whose children are experiencing rapid changes in their vision.

Mom: Cynthia
Daughter: Emily

"We noticed that he was not hitting the ball as he normally did."

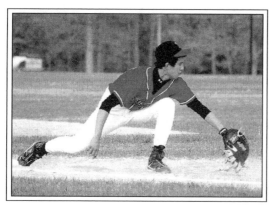

Our son Stephen has been playing baseball since he was 6 years old. At the age of 10, during the baseball season, we noticed that he was not hitting as he normally did. We took him for an eye exam and the outcome was that he needed glasses. It was hard for him adjusting to the glasses and especially wearing them during sports. One of his friends using corneal reshaping lenses recommended them. Stephen decided to give them a try and we were so glad that we did.

He started using them at the age of 11 and had absolutely no problems with this technology. He was so happy to be able to play sports without any glasses. He is now 15 and is still using corneal reshaping lenses. He plays multiple sports in high school including baseball, basketball and soccer.

Besides not having to wear glasses, we are also very happy that his vision level has not changed since he started using them.

Dad: Ken
Son: Stephen

"Today Vinaya is a happy child."

Our daughter, Vinaya, is 14 years old. We still remember that bitter, distressful day in our life when Vinaya (she was 10 at that time) came from school holding her broken eyeglasses in her hand.

Today Vinaya is a happy child. She got rid of her eyeglasses, plus the corneal reshaping seems to have hindered the further deterioration of her eyesight. Her confidence level is up.

We are profusely thankful for this technology and our doctors for their high level of commitment and care.

Parents: Srinivas & Sireesha
Daughter: Vinaya

Notes from Students

<hr />

Appendix C

<hr />

There are so many children who have successfully worn corneal reshaping lenses a good portion of their lives. They have grown up into wonderful adults we felt the need to share their stories and experiences with you.

"The eye doctor gave me back the only thing I've ever wanted...my vision."

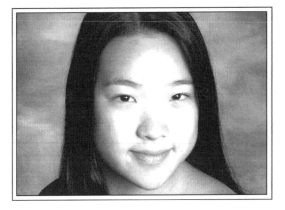

I am a certified bookworm. When I was really young, I would read books nonstop regardless of whether it was day or night, light or dark. I'd never have imagined it then, but reading books had its downside. In sixth grade, I had to get my first pair of glasses because I couldn't see anything the teacher put on the board. But even glasses didn't stop my vision from getting worse. After that initial pair I had to get four more pairs, each one stronger than the last. Every year the thickness of my glasses increased and pretty soon, my grades started dropping. By eighth grade, my vision was so bad that I literally could not see what I was typing on my computer screen without glasses. By then, I was starting to lose hope of ever being able to see again without huge, heavy glasses.

My sincerest wish was to be able to see perfectly again without glasses or contacts—and I was willing to do anything, including putting a stop to my reading—to achieve that dream.

When my mother first brought up the topic of corneal reshaping lenses I completely ignored her and shot down the idea. I was sick of contacts and glasses, and I'd given up all hope of being able to see normally again. However, my mom persisted. Now, three years later, I can honestly say that one appointment changed my whole life.

I'd never have thought it possible, but the eye doctor gave me back the only thing I've ever wanted—my vision. I could once again see perfectly in the daytime without glasses or contact lenses.

Alice

"Seven years ...I am still wearing the corneal reshaping lenses."

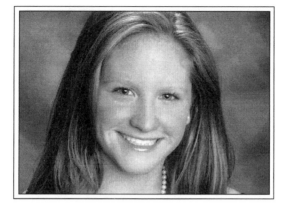

I started wearing corneal reshaping lenses when I was in sixth grade. I had glasses before that, but never wanted to wear them and it seemed that with every trip to the eye doctor, my vision was getting worse and worse.

As a competitive swimmer, I was in the pool up to eight times a week and glasses and regular contacts were both a hassle. When I wore glasses, my vision in the water was poor and I would end practice with headaches from straining my eyes. I had seen many teammates stop during practice because they had lost a contact while swimming.

My eye doctor suggested the corneal reshaping lenses. I was a little apprehensive about putting hard contacts into my eyes at night and taking them out during the day. I didn't believe that I would have perfect vision without the aid of glasses or contacts! However, I had no problems with the lenses and in a short period it became routine to put them in before I went to sleep or in the evening while reading or watching T.V. They were not uncomfortable, as I had expected, but instead were incredibly easy to get used to.

The effects that wearing the corneal reshaping lenses had on my day to day life were immediate and pronounced. Schoolwork became easier, and I didn't have to worry about losing a contact during the swim practice. I never had headaches and I really did have near perfect vision during the day.

Elizabeth

"*I started wearing corneal reshaping lenses as a teenager.*"

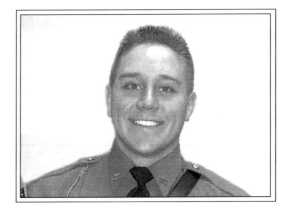

I started wearing corneal reshaping lenses as a teenager. I maintain a highly active lifestyle, which includes practicing law as an attorney, a job in law enforcement, and participating in numerous sports activities. Prior to using corneal reshaping lenses my vision was poor, affecting many facets of life. When our family eye doctor suggested trying newly introduced corneal reshaping lenses to my mother, I jumped at the opportunity.

After one day of using corneal reshaping, I realized this method matched my lifestyle perfectly. No longer did I have to rely on unwieldy glasses or bothersome soft contact lenses. Corneal reshaping enabled me to progress in my career, studies and hobbies without those burdensome apparatuses.

I recommend this technology to anyone seeking a simple, effective and non-surgical way to enhance their vision and life!

Jake

"Wearing these lenses every night has become as routine as brushing my teeth."

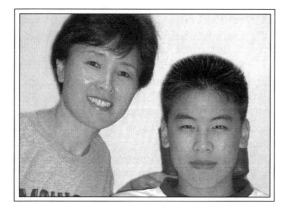

As a veteran of corneal reshaping for almost eight years, wearing these lenses every night has become as routine as brushing my teeth. However, this is not to say that corneal reshaping has not had an impact on my life. In fact, corneal reshaping may have been one of the most significant changes I went through next to going to college.

Corneal reshaping has brought my eyes from not being able to see any of the letters on an eye chart to near perfect vision within the first few days.

What convinced me to try it as a youngster was my worsening eyesight. My eyes were getting worse every year I wore eyeglasses, affecting my depth perception. Now I notice an improvement in the sports I play. It has been almost a decade since the last time I saw with poor vision.

Leo

"I won silver at the renowned Junior Olympics for Tae Kwon Do."

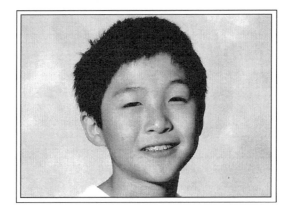

In the fast-paced sport of Tae Kwon Do, there is no time to readjust glasses in the midst of combat. Ever since I started Tae Kwon Do at the age of eight, things always seemed blurry and I could not train to my full potential. My parents decided to take a new approach, corneal reshaping lenses, after getting recommendations from the parents of my friend. They were amazing! You would only have to put them on at night, and then in the morning your eyes would see things with better clarity. At first, my natural reflexes shut my eyes every time the contact lenses came close to them, but gradually I was able to put them in easily.

After one year of wearing these lenses and four months of rigorous training, I won silver at the renowned Junior Olympics for Tae Kwon Do in 2006. Two years later, I returned to the Junior Olympics in 2008. My eyesight was sharp and precise. It seemed like magic, but I was able to predict my opponent's moves, and I countered it quickly.

During a short pause, I saw my parents cheering for me, and in a rush of power, speed, and adrenaline, I won in the last ten seconds. Can you do that with glasses?

Frank

"We both wore soft lenses."

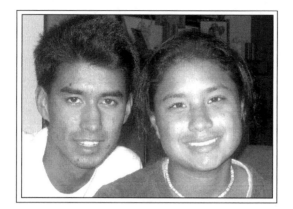

Depth perception and clarity are very important characteristics in any sport activity, especially in tennis. We both wore soft lenses. Every year, our eyeglass power would increase and it became increasingly difficult to play. Line calls from the other side of the tennis court became questionable. Also, on clay or hard surfaces using soft lenses was often a liability because of the dust or dirt getting into our eyes. Practice drills and tennis matches during windy days just made it worse, including the dryness of our eyes after a while.

After attending a lecture on corneal reshaping, we decided to give it a try. We were amazed at the results! After using the lenses for two nights, we were able to see better. Lines and balls were no longer blurred. Windy days did not bother us anymore. Now without any lenses in our eyes, we find that even sudden movements like serving in a tennis match is not that difficult. The result is that there is marked improvement in the sports that we play and even in our music performances. There are also no vision-related headaches.

We would highly recommend it to anyone looking for alternatives to soft contact lenses.

Josh and Jamila

Future Reading

―――――――― Appendix D ――――――――

This book is written for parents, it's not a scientific text, just the opinion of the authors, describing their clinical observations spanning decades.

Parents have a wide range of backgrounds and interests. So, we included a base for parents to further research the topics discussed, if they so desire. Many of the articles and books can be reviewed and purchased with relative ease through the Internet. This is not an exhaustive review of the literature, just documentation of some of the books and research discussed in our book.

1. Kurtz, D., Hyman, L., Gwiazda, J., Manny, R., Dong, L., Wang, Y., et al. (2007). Role of parental myopia in the progression of myopia and its interaction with treatment in COMET children. *Investigative Ophthalmology and Visual Science*, 48, 562-70.

2. Zadnik, K., Satariano, W., Mutti, D., Sholtz, R., & Adams, A. (1994, May). The effect of parental history of myopia in children's eye size. *The Journal of the American Medical Association*, 271, 1323-27.

3. Morgan, I., & Rose, K. (2005). How genetic is school myopia. Progress in Retinal and Eye Research, 24, 1-38.

4. Mutti, D., Mitchell, G., Moeschberger, M., Jones, L., & Zadnik, K. (2002). Parental myopia, near work, school achievement, and children's refractive error. Investigative Ophthalmology and Visual Science, 43, 3633-640.

5. Saw, S., Wu, H., Seet, B., Wong, T., Yap, E., Chia, K., et al. (2001, July). Academic achievement, close up work parameters, and myopia in Singapore military. British Journal of Ophthalmology, 85, 855-60.

6. Saw, S., Gazzard, G., Shih-Yen, E. C., Chua, W. (2005). *Myopia and associated pathological complications. Ophthalmic and Physiological Optics*, 25, 381-391.

7. Wong, T., Klein, B., Klein, R., Tomany, S., & Lee, K. (2001). Refractive errors and incident cataracts: The Beaver Dam Eye Study. *Investigative Ophthalmology and Visual Science*, 42, 1449-54.

8. Younan, C., Mitchell, P., Cumming, R., Rochtchina, E., & Wang, J. (2002). Myopia and incident cataract and cataract surgery: The Blue Mountains Eye Study. *Investigative Ophthalmology and Visual Science*, 43, 3625-32.

9. Wong, T. Y., Klein, B. E. K., Klein, R., Knudtson, M., & Lee, K. E. (2003, January). Refractive errors, intraocular pressure, and glaucoma in a white population. *Ophthalmology*, 110(1), 221-217.

10. Mitchell, P., Hourihan, F., Sandbach, J., & Jin Wang, J. (1999, October). The relationship between glaucoma and myopia. The Blue Mountains eye study. *Ophthalmology*, 106(10), 2010-15.

11. Vongphanit, J., Mitchell, P., & Jin Wang, J. (2002). Prevalence and progression of myopic retinopathy in an older population. *Ophthalmology*, 109(4), 704-11.

12. Gozum, N., Cakir, M., Gucukoglu, A., & Sezen, F. (1997). Relationship between retinal lesions and axial length, age and sex in high myopia. *European Journal of Ophthalmology*, 7(3), 277-82.

13. Wilson, A., & Woo, G. (1989, October). A review of the prevalence and causes of myopia. *Singapore Medical Journal*, 30(5), 479-84.

14. Zylbermann, R., Landau, D., & Berson, D. (1993, September/October). The influence of study habits on myopia in Jewish teenagers. *Journal of Pediatric Ophthalmology and Strabismus*, 30(5), 319-22.

15. *Asian America* [Television broadcast]. (2006, March). New York City: Public Broadcasting Service.

16. Friedman, T. (2005). *The World is Flat: A Brief History of the Twenty-first Century*. Farrar, Straus and Giroux.

17. Our view on equal education: Admission to college isn't just about grades, test scores. (2008, July 7). *USA Today*, p. A10.

18. Grosvenor, T. (2003, September). Why is there an epidemic of myopia? *Clinical and Experimental Optometry*, 86(5), 273-5.

19. Ong, E., & Ciuffreda, K. (1995). Nearwork-induced transient myopia: a critical review. *Documenta ophthalmologica. Advances in ophthalmology*, 91(1), 57-85.

20. Rose, K., Morgan, I., Kifley, A., Huynh, S., Smith, W., & Mitchell, P. (2008, August). Outdoor activity reduces the prevalence of myopia in children. *Ophthalmology*, 115(8), 1279-85.

21. Stenson, S., & Rashkind, R. (1970). Pseudomyopia: etiology, mechanisms and therapy. *Journal of Pediatric Ophthalmology and Strabismus*, 7, 110-15.

22. Rosenfield, M., & Gilmartin, B. (1998). Myopia and Nearwork. Oxford, Butterworth-Heinemann.

23. Gwiazda, J., Hyman, L., Norton, T., Hussein, M., Marsh-Tootle, W., Manny, R., et al. (2004, July). Accommodation and related risk factors associated with myopia progression and their interaction with treatment in COMET children. *Investigative Ophthalmology and Visual Science*, 45(7), 2143-151.

24. Up to 1.6 million high schoolers may have untreated vision problems. (1996, August 27). *Business Wire*.

25. Birnbaum, M. (1993). *Optometric management of near point vision disorders*. Butterworth-Heinemann.

26. Birnbaum, M. (1984). Near point visual stress: a physiological model. *Journal of the American Optometric Association*, 55, 825-35.

27. Hung, L., Ramamirtham, R.,Huang, J., Qiao-Grider, Y., & Smith, E. (2008). Peripheral Refraction in Normal Infant Rhesus Monkeys. *Investigative Ophthalmology and Visual Science*, 49(9), 3747-3757.

28. Hung, L., Crawford, M., & Smith, E. (1995). Spectacle lenses alter eye growth and the refractive status of young monkeys. *Nature Medicine*, (1), 761-65.

29. Kee, C., Hung, L., Qiao-Grider, Y., Ramamirtham, R., & Smith, E. (2005). Astigmatism in monkeys with experimentally induced myopia or hyperopia. *Optometry and Vision Science*, 46, 248-60.

30. Smith, E., Kee, C., Ramamirtham, R., Qiao-Grider, Y., & Hung, L. (2005). Peripheral vision can dominate eye growth and refractive development. *Investigative Ophthalmology and Visual Science*, 46, 3965-72.

31. Chung, K., Mohidin, N., & O'Leary, D. (2002, October). Undercorrection of myopia enhances rather than inhibits myopia progression. *Vision Research*, 42(22), 2555-559.

32. Wildsoet, C., & Norton, T. (1999, June). Toward controlling myopia progression? *Optometry and Vision Science*, 76(6), 341-42.

33. Drexler, W., Findl, O., Schmetterer, L., Hitzenberger, C., & Fercher, A. (1998, October). Eye elongation during accommodation in humans: differences between emmetropes and myopes. *Investigative Ophthalmology and Visual Science*, (11), 2140-47.

34. Mallen, E. (2006, March). Transient axial length change during the accommodation response in young adults. *Investigative Ophthalmology and Visual Science*, 47(3), 1251-54.

35. Shum, P., Ko, L., Ng, C., & Lin, S. (1993, January). A biometric study of ocular changes during accommodation. *American Journal of Ophthalmology*, 115(1), 76-81.

36. Daubs, J. (1984). Some geographic, environmental and nutritive concomitants of malignant myopia. *Ophthalmic and Physiological Optics*, 4(2), 143-49.

37. Fulk, G., Cyert, L., & Parker, D. (2002, January). Seasonal variation in myopia progression and ocular elongation. *Optometry and Vision Science*, 79(1), 46-51.

38. Goss, D., & Rainey, B. (1998). Relation of childhood myopia progression rates to time of year. *Journal of the American Optometric Association*, 69, 262-66.

39. Chiu, C.-J., Hubbard, L. D., Armstrong, J., Rogers, G., Jacques, P. F., Chylack, L. T., Jr., et al. (2006, April). Dietary glycemic index and carbohydrate in relation to early age-related macular degeneration. *American Journal of Clinical Nutrition*, 83(4), 880-86.

40. Chiu, C.-J., Milton, R. C., Gensler, G., & Taylor, A. (2006, May). Dietary carbohydrate intake and glycemic index in relation to cortical and nuclear lens opacities in the Age-Related Eye Disease Study. *American Journal of Clinical Nutrition*, 83(5), 1177-84.

41. Richer, S. (2005, December). Put your patients on the pyramid. *Review of Optometry*, 142(12).

42. Schmid, K. (2008). Myopia Manual. An Impartial Documentation of all Reasons, Therapies and Recommendations. PageFree Publishing, Inc.

43. Walsh, B. (2008, June 23). It's not just genetics. *Time*, 70-80.

44. US Department of Health and Human Services & US Department of Agriculture. (2005). *Dietary Guidelines for Americans, 2005* (6th ed.). Washington, DC: US Government Printing Office.

45. McBrien, N., & Gentle, A. (2003, May). Role of the sclera in the development and pathological complications of myopia. *Progress in Retinal and Eye Research*, 22(3), 307-38.

46. Rada, J., Shelton, S., & Norton, T. (2005, September). The sclera and myopia. *Experimental Eye Research,* 82 (2), 185-200.

47. Cordain, L., Eaton, S., Brand Miller, J., Lindeberg, S., & Jensen, C. (2002, April). An evolutionary analysis of the etiology and pathogenesis of juvenile onset myopia. *Acta Ophthalmologica Scandinavica,* 80(20), 125-35.

48. Cordain, L., Eades, M., & Eades, M. (2003, September). Hyperinsulinemic diseases of civilization: more than just Syndrome X. *Comparative Biochemistry and Physiology,* 136(1), 95-112.

49. Chua, W., Balakrishnan, V., Chan, Y., Tong, L., Ling, Y., Quah, B., et al. (n.d.). Atropine for the treatment of childhood myopia. *Ophthalmology,* 113(12), 2285-91.

50. Shih, Y., Chen, C., Chou, A., Ho, T., Lin, L., & Hung, P. (1999, February). Effects of different concentrations of atropine on controlling myopia in myopic children. *Journal of Ocular Pharmacology and Therapeutics,* 15(1), 85-90.

51. Yen, M., Liu, J., Kao, S., & Shiao, C. (1989, May). Comparison of the effect of atropine and cyclopentolate on myopia. *Annals of Ophthalmology,* 21(5), 180-2, 187.

52. Luft, W, Ming, Y, Stell, W. (2003, March). Variable effects of previously untested muscarinic receptor antagonists on experimental myopia. *Investigative Ophthalmology and Visual Science;* 44(3), 1330-8.

53. Lee, J., Fang, P., Yang, I., Chen, C., Lin, P., Lin, S., et al. (2006, February). Prevention of myopia progression with 0.05% atropine solution. *Journal of Ocular Pharmacology and Therapeutics,* 22(1), 41-6.

54. Adler, D., & Millodot, M. (2006, September). The possible effect of undercorrection on myopic progression in children. *Clinical and Experimental Optometry,* 89(5), 315-21.

55. Gwiazda, J. E., Hyman, L., Norton, T. T., Hussein, M. E., Marsh-Tootle, W., Manny, R., et al. (2004). Accommodation and related risk factors associated with myopia progression and their interaction with treatment in COMET children. *Invest Ophthalmol Vis Sci,* 45(7), 2143-2151.

56. Hastings Edwards, M., Wing-Hong Li, R., Siu-yin Lam, C., Kwok-fai Lew, J., & Sin-ying Yu, B. (2002, September). The Hong Kong progressive lens myopia control study: Study design and Main findings. *Investigative Ophthalmology and Visual Science,* 43(9), 2852-858.

57. Fulk, G., Cyert, L., & Parker, D. (2000, August). A randomized trial of the effect of single vision vs. bifocal lenses on myopia progression in children with esophoria. *Optometry and Vision Science,* 77(8), 395-401.

58. Gwiazda, J., Hyman, L., Hussein, M., Everett, D., Norton, T., Kurtz, D., et al. (2003, April). A randomized clinical trial of progressive addition lenses versus single vision lenses on the progression of myopia in children. *Investigative Ophthalmology and Visual Science,* 44(4), 1492-500.

59. LASIK eye surgery: *What are the risks and how can I find the right doctor for me?* (n.d.). Retrieved October 21, 2008, from http://www.fda.gov/cdrh/lasik/risks.htm

60. Walline, J. (2007, September). Contact Lenses In Pediatrics (CLIP) study: Chair time and ocular health. *Optometry and Vision Science*, 84(9), 896-902.

61. Walline, J., Jones, L., Sinnott, L., Manny, R., Gaume, A., Rah, M., et al. (2008, June). A randomized trial of the effect of soft contact lenses on myopia progression in children. *Investigative Ophthalmology and Visual Science*.

62. Walline, J., Jones, L., Mutti, D., & Zadnik, K. (2004, December). A randomized trial of the effects of rigid contact lenses on myopia progression. *Archives of Ophthalmology*, 122(12), 1760-766.

63. Katz, J., Schein, O., Levy, B., Cruiscullo, T., Saw, S., Rajan, U., et al. (2003, July). A randomized trial to assess the impact of rigid gas permeable contact lenses on progression of children's myopia. *American Journal of Ophthalmology*, 136(1), 82-90.

64. Walline, J., Jones, L., Chitkara, M., Coffey, B., Jackson, J., Manny, R., et al. (2006, January). The adolescent and child health initiative to encourage vision empowerment (ACHIEVE) study design and baseline data. *Optometry and Vision Science*, 83(1), 37-45.

65. Holden, B. (2004). The myopia epidemic: Is there a role for corneal refractive therapy? *Eye and Contact Lens*, 4, 244-46.

66. Reim, T., Lund, M., & Wu, R. (2003, March). Orthokeratology and adolescent myopia control. *Contact Lens Spectrum*, 40-42.

67. Cho, P., Cheung, S. W., & Edwards, M. (2005). The Longitudinal Orthokeratology Research in Children (LORIC) in Hong Kong: A pilot study on refractive changes and myopia control. *Current Eye Research*, 30, 71-80.

68. Walline, J. (2007, October). *Corneal Reshaping and Yearly Observations Of Nearsightedness (CRAYON) two year results.* Lecture presented at American Academy of Optometry meeting, Tampa, FL.

69. Walline, J. (2007, June). Slowing myopia progression with lenses: Corneal reshaping may be a future alternative for slowing myopia progression in children. *Contact Lens Spectrum*, 22-27.

70 .Walline, J., Holden, B., Bullimore, M., Rah, M., Asbell, P., Barr, J., et al. (2005, September). The current state of corneal reshaping. *Eye and Contact Lens*, 31(5), 209-14.

71. Walline, J., Rah, M., & Jones, L. (2004, June). The Children's Overnight Orthokeratology Investigation (COOKI) pilot study. *Optometry and Vision Science*, 81(6), 407-13.

Getting Started

This section was designed to provide parents with a step-by-step outline and place to record the necessary information required when determining if corneal reshaping is right for your child. If you decide to proceed, it will also aid you in organizing future appointments.

1. Have your child's eyes examined for the following things:
   a. Eye health structures
   b. Nearsightedness (myopia)
   c. Farsightedness (hyperopia)
   d. Astigmatism

2. If your child has myopia or astigmatism, locate a corneal reshaping specialist:
   a. Ask a friend / eye doctor or a referral
   b. www.Bausch.com
   c. www.Ortho-K.net
   d. www.OKGlobal.org
   e. www.ParagonCRT.com

3. Prior to the consultation – DO YOUR HOMEWORK:
   a. Visit the eye doctor's website
   b. Gather information about the office
   c. Make sure your child is on board and excited!

4. You should bring the following things with you to the initial consultation:
   a. Your child's eyeglasses (if applicable)
   b. Most recent eye exam records
   c. List of questions for the eye doctor

5. Some good questions to ask are:
   a. How do you determine if my child can wear corneal reshaping lenses?
   b. How long have you been fitting children?
   c. What side effects can be expected?
   d. What do the fees include?
   e. How often do you normally adjust the fit; once, twice, etc.?
   f. Is a spare pair of lenses included?
   g. Are you comfortable working with more than one lens design?
   h. Do you have a refund policy?
   i. How many appointments are typically required?

—— My Child's Corneal Reshaping Diary ——

Consultation Appointment:

Some offices require you to bring both your child's eyeglasses as well as a copy of the most recent eye exam with you to this appointment.

Some good questions to ask the doctor are:

1. How do you determine if my child can wear corneal reshaping lenses?

_____

_____

_____

2. How long have you been fitting children?

_____

_____

_____

3. What side effects can be expected?

_____

_____

_____

4. How many appointments are typically required the first year? The second year, etc.?

_____

_____

_____

5. What do the fees include?

_____

_____

_____

6. How often do you normally adjust the fit; once, twice, etc.?

_____

_____

_____

7. Is a spare pair of lenses included?

_____

_____

_____

8. Do you have a refund policy?

_____

_____

_____

9. Are you comfortable working with more than one lens design?

_____

_____

_____

Future Appointments

	Date	Notes from Appointment
Appointment 1		
Appointment 2		
Appointment 3		
Appointment 4		
Appointment 5		
Appointment 6		
Appointment 7		
Appointment 8		

2518246

Made in the USA